THE SECRET
OF THE NON DIET

RUDY KACHMANN, M.D. · KIM KACHMANN-GELTZ

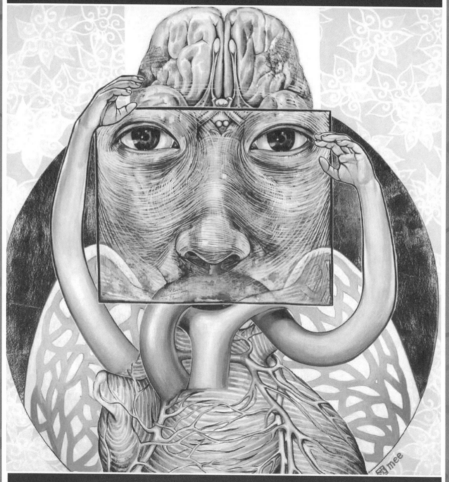

How to restore energy, lose weight, avoid and reverse chronic
diseases, look good and feel good WITHOUT DIETING.

Published by Rudy Kachmann, M.D. Kachmann Media, LLC
www.KachmannMindBody.com

Library of Congress Control Number: 2009924297

ISBN-10: 0-9823957-0-1
ISBN-13: 978-0-9823957-0-7

Printed in the United States of America

CONTENTS

NOTE TO THE READER

The advice we offer in this book should supplement, not supplant, the advice of your personal physician. Changes in your diet or exercise regime may require medical supervision if you are pregnant, or are a patient with a chronic illness. Following the dietary and lifestyle suggestions in this book could impact the effect of certain types of medication. Before taking new vitamins or supplements, be sure to consult with your doctor. The authors and publisher disclaim any liability directly, or indirectly, from the use of the material in this book by any person.

The stories we tell are true. Certain details, however, have been changed to protect patient confidentiality and privacy.

PREFACE

Neurosurgeons and neurologists like to joke that cardiologists have hijacked atherosclerosis, the clinical term for artery disease, and put the spotlight on the heart, a multi-billion-dollar medical business. Almost 10 percent of the increase in U.S. health care spending over the past decade was due to angioplasty and stenting, the surgery to clear blood vessels. But, atherosclerosis attacks the entire circulatory system, affecting every vital organ, especially the brain, which is my area of business. Strokes are the number one cause of disability and third leading cause of death in the U.S. For the sake of simplicity, and to emphasize that atherosclerosis is a systemic disease that affects more than the heart, we refer to the illness as "vascular disease." It is a dynamic inflammatory process that damages blood vessels and threatens blood flow to the legs and the body's most vital organs—the brain, the kidneys and the heart.

Deaths related to vascular disease have declined sharply in the last few decades. This is thanks to revolutionary advancements in medicine: the invention of angiography to see inside the arteries of the brain and the heart; the first open-heart surgery and transplant; bypass surgery to detour blood around a blockage, or angioplasty and stenting to clear a blockage; and the development of statins, cholesterol-lowering drugs to dissolve plaque. Stem-cell research may usher in a new age of advancements—if Americans can agree to fund it.

With all our cutting-edge technology and powerful drugs, and despite the sharp decline in the death rate, half of all Americans still die of vascular disease, often before reaching age 30. Every year more than a million Americans suffer heart attacks, and almost as many more million suffer strokes—a life-changing, irreversible injury that may result in serious disabilities. Brain and heart cells cannot regenerate to any significant extent.

I believe in Medicine's capacity to triumph over the challenges presented by a life-threatening injury or acute pathology. We cannot, however, save the hearts and minds of Americans from vascular disease unless we change our focus from prescriptions and procedures to prevention and wellness. Our country performs three times as many invasive cardiac procedures, in comparison to other developed countries, but still has one of the highest death rates from vascular disease in the world. An estimated 71 million Americans suffer from heart disease, and 2.4 million die from it each year.[1]

If there's anything I've learned over the last 40 years as a physician and neurosurgeon, it's that vascular disease is dynamic. Even the "clean" arteries used in bypassing a blocked artery can become clogged in a matter of months. We also have higher rates of obesity, diabetes, cancer and high blood pressure in comparison to the rest of the world. The Centers for Disease Control and Prevention (CDC) reported in 2008 that 24 million Americans have diabetes, and increase of three million over two years. As we continue to get fatter and sicker over the next few decades, the recent drop in vascular disease deaths may slow, stop or even backslide. Yet, the disease need not exist; it is preventable.

Dr. Walter Willett, chairman of the Harvard School of Public Health's department of nutrition, and the architect of the Nurses' Health Study, one of the largest prospective studies of risk factors for chronic disease in women, suggested that better lifestyles habits could prevent 80 percent of heart disease and 90 percent of type 2 diabetes. These estimates are based on the Nurses' study and dozens of other studies focusing on the effects of lifestyle on heart disease and diabetes.

One of the most obvious but underutilized weapons in our healing arsenal is nutritional therapy, not drugs or surgery and not dieting, which implies deprivation. The No-Dieting program is a targeted nutritional strategy that leverages our bodies' efficient metabolism of whole grains, complex carbohydrates, vegetables, legumes and fruit. Metabolism determines how quickly we lose or gain weight. It involves a complex network of biochemicals that not only convert food into fuel, but also affect how efficiently we burn that fuel.

The average American's obsession with dieting and their shift away from fuel-burning complex carbohydrates has undermined their metabolism, health and permanent weight loss. Low-carb diets allow steak, eggs and other high-fat foods, do not distinguish the "good" fats from the "bad" fats, and have led to a diet that's way too high in artery-clogging saturated fats and cholesterol. Americans consume 40-50 percent of calories as fat. The link between saturated fat and vascular disease is well established. Heart attacks are almost unknown in rural Chinese villages because starchy low-fat rice, vegetables and soybeans are the dominant food staples. The Chinese use meat as a flavor enhancer for their many vegetables.

The Secret of Resistant Starch

The primary macronutrients in the foods we eat are carbohydrates, fats and protein. Contrary to popular belief, complex carbohydrates, including whole wheat pasta, bread, beans and potatoes, are not fattening. These vegetarian foods are very low in fat, high in fiber and have almost no cholesterol. And they resist digestion: we lose 30-40 percent of the calories from starchy complex carbohydrates while metabolizing. The complex carbohydrates highlighted in the No-Dieting program compliment, not battle, our biological destiny.

We haven't evolved to efficiently metabolize the processed and refined foods sold in our supermarkets. Simple carbohydrates, such as white bread, are empty calories. The process of refining bread robs almost 30 nutrients from the flour. "Enriching" flour only adds an average of four nutrients back to the bread. White bread contains few nutrients, a low percentage of whole grains and lots of sugar. It is easily converted to fat, while complex carbohydrates are rarely converted to fat by our bodies. White bread is basically sugar that you can sink your teeth into.

Refined foods contain less water and fiber, and more added fat and sugar than fresh foods. This makes them less filling, more fattening and prone to raise blood glucose and insulin, which can lead to Type 2 diabetes and vascular disease. Switching from highly refined to whole grain breads and cereals is one way to improve your odds against these diseases.

The health impact of processed and refined foods doesn't hinder the food industry from spending $30 billion annually to market them. Michael Pollan, author and columnist for the *New York Times*, recommends that if there are more than five ingredients, or you can't pronounce two or three of the ingredients, then it's not real food. It's something else. And that "something else" is making us sick.

The Standard American Diet (SAD)

For dinner, the Standard American Diet (SAD) includes a generous portion of beef, gravy, deep-fried and salted potatoes, vegetables saturated in butter or cheese, and a rich dessert. The venerable potato is often on the dinner table, but the health benefits of this starchy vegetable are often marred by butter, sour-cream or a fryer full of lard. The amount of animal protein, saturated fat, salt and sugar in our SAD diet is double, triple and sometimes even quadruple the amount required in a single meal. Consuming the SAD diet day after day raises blood pressure, blood sugar, cholesterol and triggers inflammatory mechanisms known to influence the development of obesity, diabetes, hypertension, vascular disease and common cancers. Simple changes such as replacing low fiber cereals with a 100 percent whole grain cereal; replacing white rice and potatoes with brown rice and other whole grains; and eating more fruits and vegetables can make a difference in your odds of becoming a disease statistic.

Over the past few decades, as the number of overweight patients increased sharply, my consciousness and knowledge about nutrition and diet-related disease grew. Carrying around extra weight can damage spinal discs and cause strokes and brain aneurysms, my area of business. Finally, my daughter and I decided to write a book that would show readers how to use the metabolizing of food to lose weight, prevent disease and most of all—reverse the pathological process driving vascular disease. Food can be medicine or food can be toxic.

I look at weight and poor health as a complex "mind-body problem" involving metabolism, inflammation, and the brain and nervous system. Hormones, neurotransmitters, nutrients, and cytokines—proteins produced by the immune system that control inflammation—are just some of the fundamental biological factors at play in diet-related disease. A relay of metabolic signals between the brain and the body regulates how well we recruit and use energy, and gain or lose weight. Disease and obesity occur when the communication breaks down.

For example, diet affects insulin, a fundamental hormone with multiple roles. Most digested food enters the bloodstream as sugar (glucose), the body's main source of fuel. Insulin secreted by the pancreas moves the glucose from the bloodstream into cells for fuel and prompts the liver to convert excess glucose into fat cells. Fat cells then release leptin—another fundamental hormone—to signal the brain to stop the behavior of eating. This takes place on a subconscious level.

Diabetes results when the body cannot use insulin or produces too little insulin, resulting in chronically high glucose levels that damage the body, especially the delicate endothelial cells lining arteries. Type 1 diabetes, which is typically diagnosed at an early age, occurs when the immune system mistakenly destroys cells that produce insulin. In Type 2 diabetes, which is much more common among sedentary and overweight adults, the body is resistant to the effects of insulin.

Soft drinks, rich desserts and other sugary foods sharply raise blood glucose levels and prompt the pancreas to release a surge of insulin to restore the glucose to a normal level. The sudden drop in glucose then triggers hunger signals in the brain, and off to the refrigerator we go, again and again as the cycle repeats itself. Consuming too many calories keeps insulin levels high and may eventually damage pancreatic cells, resulting in diabetes or pre-diabetes—the most common risk factor for heart attack and stroke. Management of insulin and glucose levels through diet and exercise or medication is a critical piece in the prevention of chronic diseases.

Excess weight endangers your health by raising the risk of numerous health problems. Researchers are now saying that visceral fat, which grows in and around internal organs, releases fatty acids that promote inflammation and further decreases sensitivity to insulin. In other words, not only do rich, refined foods promote insulin resistance, the weight gained contributes to the disease process. In fact, obesity raises the risk of vascular disease by 300 percent.

Diabetes Epidemic
About 95 percent of diabetes cases are Type 2, according to the Centers for Disease Control and Prevention (CDC). The total number of Americans with diabetes has grown to approximately 24 million, or 8 percent of the U.S. population, the most overt sign that as a nation, we are overloading the body with too many calories.

A Mind-Body Approach

This book approaches weight and disease from an integrative "mind-body" perspective. A common tendency, especially in the United States, is to overrate the influence of genetics, and underrate the affect of lifestyle. If your mom or dad carried extra weight around their hips or thighs, then you may do the same. Genes may influence the likelihood of developing weight in a certain area of your body, but fat genes are not *hardwired* into your chromosomes. Fat genes can be turned ON or turned OFF by how you live. Different types of foods interact with your genes leading to remarkably different effects.

Complex carbohydrates burn fat and satiate appetite. Low-carbohydrate diets ultimately end in failure because they go against the grain of our ancient biology. Fat and protein reduce the appetite very little.

This book is for the chronic dieters, people with pre-diabetes or insulin resistance, diabetes, hypertension or severe vascular disease, and those who cannot shed those extra pounds. Readers who follow the No-Dieting program will melt away fat and plaque and begin to feel better. We don't ask you to restrict calories. You will never feel deprived or hungry. We offer three different programs in which you can choose a conservative, moderate or liberal approach, depending on your weight-loss or health needs. Extreme problems will require extreme changes. If you're awaiting heart bypass, facing a second or third stent from severe coronary artery disease, or losing sensation in your feet due to unrelenting diabetes, you may want to skip to Chapter 4 and get started on the program.

Two of every three Americans are overweight—an epidemic that's spawned hundreds of diets and prompted us to spend more than $1 billion on weight-loss products each year. Even if weight or illness is not one of your problems, the No-Dieting approach to nutrition is still critically important to your continued health and wellness. More than half of the leading causes of death are driven by lifestyle factors: how we think and move, what we eat, the quality of our personal relationships, and how we cope with stress. Medicine can only do so much—the rest is up to you. I've had to teach many of my patients to reorient their thinking away from white coats and stethoscopes and onto the journey of self-care.

The "EASY" button doesn't work. You're more likely to make challenging lifestyle changes if your emotional needs are met. So I encourage you to embark on the journey towards better health with someone who supports you—a spouse, friend, partner, parent, older child or counselor. Give us six weeks. You'll become more and more motivated to change when you see and feel your body changing. Your life, and your loved ones, depend on what you are willing to do for your health. Our goal is to empower people of all ages with information and action items that could prolong or even save their life, or the life of a loved one.

Rudy Kachmann, M.D. & Kim Kachmann-Geltz, M.A.

INTRODUCTION:
How to Lose Weight and Gain Optimal Health (without Dieting)

Good news—you don't need a diet. A seemingly infinite array of diets—detox, low-carb, no-carb, high protein, Mediterranean or beach-based is flooding the marketplace. Many scientific studies have shown that deprivation diets invariably lower the body's basal metabolic rate as it struggles to conserve energy. The No-Dieting secret is how to improve your body's metabolism by increasing your consumption of complex carbohydrates—yams, corn, potatoes and many other unrefined starchy foods. Our program will help you lose weight and prevent common cancers, heart attack and stroke, or reverse metabolic syndrome, diabetes and severe vascular disease. Do you want greater vitality and optimal health? Then read on.

In my 40 years of treating the ravages of vascular disease—stroke, aneurysms, disabilities, sudden death—the hundreds of patients who followed my No-dieting program were able to lose weight and reverse chronic diseases without life-threatening surgery, or the side-effects of powerful medications. Some patients were not able to avoid surgery to prevent a second or third stroke. But my patient Diane Yardley is one of my favorite No-Dieting success stories.

Diane was a 54-year-old mechanical engineer, a pioneer in her field who led several high profile waterworks projects for the city. She had a doctorate in engineering from Purdue University and two teenagers—a fourteen-year-old boy and a seventeen-year-old girl. Like far too many middle-age Americans, Diane had gained about 5-10 pounds each year since high school, and now tipped the scales at 220 pounds. With a height of 5 feet 6 inches, Diane had a Body Mass Index (BMI) of 35 and was considered obese by medical standards: a perilously heavy weight causing life-threatening ailments, including hypertension. Her blood pressure had been dangerously high for several years at 210 over 125, but she chose to believe that it would only become a problem in the distant future.

For five years, Diane had experienced what she called "spells" in her ability to plan ahead, evaluate complicated situations at work, and multitask—shift her attention from one thing to another. I suspected that her "spells" were actually tiny strokes or transient ischemic attacks

(TIAs). I ordered an ultrasound of her carotid arteries, the large blood vessels on either side of the neck that supply blood to the brain. The carotid arteries nourish the front part of the brain where thinking, planning and other important functions are thought to reside.

I also ordered a full lipid-panel to analyze her cholesterol levels. Diane's LDL, "bad" cholesterol, was too high at 240. I set a goal to lower her LDL to less than 80, and raise her HDL to greater than 45. Her imaging scan revealed severe carotid stenosis—more than 70 percent blockage of the left carotid artery, a severe buildup of fat and cholesterol deposits called plaque. Her second image from a CTA (Computer Tomography Angiogram) that uses injected dye to produce more detailed images inside veins and arteries, revealed that her left frontal lobe had several small areas of ischemic tissue. Blood flow to a critical area of the brain was blocked—the frontal lobes are thought to be the part of the brain where executive functions reside.

The results of Diane's tests made her "spells" make sense: the accumulation of mini strokes, ischemic tissue, and blockage in her neck artery were causing sporadic episodes of brain fog. Diane was suffering from severe vascular disease and was at high risk for a full-blown stroke, or even a heart attack. Vascular disease is systemic; if severe plaque is found in one artery, then more than likely it will be present in the arteries feeding the heart, legs and brain.

Taking Action

Diane was an apt listener as I described our urgent plan of action which included aspirin therapy and blood pressure medication. Unlike few physicians today, I spent an hour going over critical lifestyle changes, including the three phases of my No-Dieting nutrition plan. No one gains weight overnight. Most people gain weight and become sick so gradually that they can't figure out how it happened. Like most of my patients who are overweight and sick, Diane also didn't know how to quit dieting. I asked her if she wanted to be permanently thin or only temporarily thin. Diets are temporary measures with temporary results. Dieting forces our mind and body to adapt to deprivation which often becomes a vicious cycle of food denial, followed by food binges. Changing how you understand and look at food will lead to permanent weight loss and better health. But changing how you think is the first step: healthy thinking leads to healthful living.

Health problems cannot be solved by medical technology alone. A variety of behavioral, environmental and genetic factors determine well-being, but none are more important than how you think. Unless you are dependent on another human being for your care, only you will select the foods you eat, decide whether or not to exercise, quit smoking and better manage stress.

Diane seemed committed to the program, and began to exercise daily. After three months, she returned to my practice and reported no new "spells." She also had lost 10 pounds. A year later, her brain fog was a distant memory, and she had dropped a dramatic 70 pounds. Her face was radiant but her cheeks were no longer flushed—a sign that her blood pressure had returned to normal. In fact, Diane was able to quit taking her blood pressure medication, but continued on aspirin therapy as a woman with a lifelong disease. I ordered another ultrasound to check the diseased artery and compared it to the image from a year ago. The plaque in the artery had reversed to the extent that she would not require stenting or an endarterectomy, a potentially life-threatening procedure to clear a severely blocked carotid artery.

Obesity—over 100 pounds of excess weight—reduces life expectancy by 75 percent. Diane is one of hundreds of patients with progressive vascular disease who responded dramatically to simple, life-saving changes in nutrition, exercise, and relaxation techniques. She is living proof that the No-Dieting program works.

The New View of Vascular Disease

Surprising new evidence shows that nearly half of all sudden deaths, heart attacks and strokes occur without warning. The silent perpetrator is inflammation festering in a variety of hidden places throughout the body, including the belly. About 50 percent of people who die from vascular complications have abnormal cardiac markers. The other 50 percent of victims have normal cholesterol levels, but high levels of inflammation.

Abdominal fat is one of the main underlying causes of chronic inflammation that drives weight gain, diabetes, vascular disease and even cancer. Measuring your waist size is a good gauge of whether you've got too much belly fat. For women, your waist size should be 35 inches or less. For men, your waist size should not exceed 40 inches.

Vascular disease is the leading cause of death for both men and women in the U.S.[2] For most of the 20th century, doctors compared the disease to a plumbing problem. Too much cholesterol built-up in arteries, clogging them over time like corrosion in a pipe until one day, a total blockage would occur, causing a heart attack or stroke. Today we know that the immune system's reaction to the fatty build-up—not the culmination of plaque— causes 95 percent of all strokes and heart attacks.

The identification of inflammation as the main culprit in vascular disease is one of the major shifts taking place in the medical community today. Eric Topol, M.D., Chairman of the Cleveland Clinic Heart Center, said the new information about inflammation, "changes everything."[3] As our medical knowledge has grown, the goals of prevention and treatment have changed, but not fast enough. An estimated 30 million "healthy" middle-age Americans may have high levels of silent inflammation, putting them at risk for serious disability or premature death.[4] The CDC estimates that each year, a half a million Americans die from vascular disease with no prior warning.

Lowering cholesterol, especially the "bad" LDL cholesterol, with statins is beneficial but not enough. And opening a blocked artery with clot-busting drugs, balloons or stents may be lifesaving in the early hours after a stroke or heart attack, but devices don't reduce the risk of future events. Angioplasty with stenting helps symptoms, but does not cure the fundamental cause of vascular disease. Targeting inflammation generated by visceral fat, insulin resistance and Type 2 diabetes are more urgent and relative objectives in this day and age.

Think Prevention, Not Intervention
A study involving 2,280 patients reported in the New England Journal of Medicine in March of 2007, found that the use of medication, angioplasty, and stenting provides no long-term advantage over a preventive plan that include proper diagnosis, medication and lifestyle improvements.

The new view of vascular disease stems from a better understanding of how the immune system functions, in health and illness. One of the frontier areas is the link between vascular inflammation and the foods we eat, the focus of this book. Our immune system, programmed to identify and purge outside invaders like bacteria and viruses, can also be triggered by the toxins of cigarette smoke, the biochemicals of stress, and diet. These factors cause the release of chemicals, and the activation of cells involved in the inflammatory process, that lead to plaque and the formation of blood clots. Inflammation drives vascular disease from the development of fatty plaques in the walls of arteries to the rupture of those plaques.

When too much LDL cholesterol enters the bloodstream, it seeps between the tissue layers of arteries, triggering an inflammatory response that festers and damages the blood vessel with pimple-like plaques. A key inflammatory marker, called C-reactive protein (CRP), also rises. Arteries produce CRP at sites where there is cholesterol buildup. Doctors can measure vascular inflammation with an inexpensive, but highly sensitive blood test called hsCRP.

Healthy arteries function like hollow, elastic tubes that allow blood to course through all of the twists and turns of the circulatory system. Their job is to take oxygen-rich blood away from the heart and deliver it to other vital organs. Plaque changes the biology of the artery, reducing its capacity to dilate and constrict under normal physical or emotional stress, reducing blood flow. The result is often lasting damage to the heart, legs, brain and kidneys. An increase in arterial stiffness of the kidneys' arteries impairs their ability to rid the body of salt and water, increasing blood pressure and the risk of brain aneurysms and heart failure. Accumulations of plaque in the cerebral arteries leading to the brain not only predisposes to stroke, but also dementia and Alzheimer's disease.

No Warning Bell
The first symptom of heart disease in 50% of victims is sudden cardiac death.

Plaques can begin as early as primary school from genetic and lifestyle factors, and may grow denser each year without intervention. Inflammation at a young age can be caused by childhood diseases such as arthritis or diabetes, tobacco use and even high blood pressure or cholesterol. It is not uncommon to find an American teenager with high cholesterol. Even a lack of exercise has been proven to raise inflammation and increase vascular risk. Johns Hopkins researcher Samia Mora, M.D. found that as CRP levels went up, fitness levels went down.[5]

Older, calcified plaques tend to be larger, but more stable than festering, "vulnerable" plaques that have soft lipid cores. Vulnerable plaques resemble pus-filled pimples and may be anywhere in the arterial wall, not just where a blockage has formed from the buildup of plaque. And they often go undetected by angiography, the X-ray examination of blood vessels. A soft-plaque can tear or rupture, and trigger rapid clotting that blocks blood-flow to the brain or heart muscle in seconds as blood cells clump together to try to repair the artery.

During a stroke or heart attack, cells in the brain or heart muscle die from oxygen starvation, leaving scar tissue. With the advent of magnetic resonance imaging (MRI), radiologists can see detailed images of the heart or brain that reveal dead tissue—areas that have lost blood flow. If enough scar tissue develops in the heart, the muscle stiffens and can no longer pump blood to organs and tissues effectively. The symptoms of congestive heart failure ensue, along with a significant drop in the quality of life. A large stroke may result in permanent paralysis, speech impairments or other serious neurological deficits. The U.S. spends an estimated $40 billion a year caring for the disabled victims of stroke.

Vascular disease is a dynamic inflammatory process with cycles of injury, healing and re-injury. Diet plays a vital role in vascular health, and can have striking effects on inflammation and the progression of plaque.

How We Organized This Book

We organized *The Non-Diet Secrets* into two main sections. In Part I, we discuss the three main nutrients—carbohydrates, fats, and protein—and how they are digested, metabolized and stored by the body. We will teach you the secrets of working with your body's metabolism, not against it, to lose weight and reverse illness. For readers interested in finding recipes and menus that follow the principles of the No-Dieting, please turn to our "Recommended Reading List" at the end of the book.

We don't like to use the word "diet" because it sounds restrictive. The scientifically-based No-Dieting plan won't make you feel hungry. After presenting the No-Dieting secrets, we offer flexitarian, vegan and vegetarian prescription that you can tailor to your particular needs. For example, patients who are facing a second or third balloon or stent to stave-off a heart attack, may want to get started with the vegan prescription. Vegans don't eat meat or dairy products. An obese patient with several risk factors for vascular disease, such as diabetes and hypertension, should follow the vegetarian plan, and can expect to lose 5-15 pounds each month. Nutrient-dense foods, which also leverage metabolism, have the power to melt away pounds and reverse the plaque of vascular disease. Our prescriptions are based on my clinical experience and the scientific studies cited throughout the book.

Knowing that human beings aren't perfect, we also follow the 10 percent rule: 80-90 percent of what you consume must follow the No-Dieting program in order to have an impact on your weight or health. The remaining percentage is wiggle room. You may enjoy an unexpected treat, a piece of birthday cake, and so on. Vegetarians can consume dairy products, but we recommend no-fat dairy. A flexitarian prescription was designed for the healthy person who wants to remain that way. Flexitarians can eat poultry and fish on occasion, but must avoid red meat which is high in artery-clogging fat. This way of eating will help prevent common diseases and slow the rate of aging. Chapter 4 explains the scientific rationale for the plans.

In Part II, we explore the old myths and new insights into vascular disease and the top risk markers: inflammation, cholesterol, metabolic syndrome, diabetes, hypertension, obesity, smoking, aerobic fitness and stress. Our approach emphasizes the relationship between health and behavior—the mind-body connection and the circuit of communication between the heart and the brain. One of the first steps for anyone interested in reversing the odds of vascular disease is to assess their risk factors. Your risk grows with each factor. Multiple factors mean a much higher risk level. Every American can take steps to lower their risk of stroke and heart attack by addressing these risk factors. Control of risk factors is especially critical for patients who already have vascular disease.

Diet-related Disease

Disease, disability and death often begin in the digestive system, starting with what we put in our mouths. Many studies prove that nutrition makes the biggest difference in terms of disease prevention and a long lifespan. The saturated fats in meat, milk and cheese are caustic; they boost the liver's production of artery-clogging LDL cholesterol. Doctors and scientists are only beginning to understanding the health impact of the added ingredients in processed foods: artificial sweeteners, bleaching agents, high-fructose corn syrup, preservatives, sodium, hydrogenated or partially-hydrogenated oils and many others.

About 75 percent of the earth's population, primarily non-Western cultures, that consume a traditional diet of natural foods, rarely experience vascular disease and diet-related cancers, according to the most comprehensive study on nutrition and disease ever conducted: The China Study. Cornell University nutritional biochemist, T. Colin Campbell, Ph.D., led a survey of Chinese death rates for more than 2,400 counties and 880 million, or 96 percent, of their citizens over a 20 year period. Oxford University and the Chinese Academy of Preventive Medicine also conducted the project. One of the questions they explored was why the Chinese in rural villages, where food customs had not changed in centuries, enjoyed low rates of cancer and vascular disease while the urban Chinese were as sick as their Western counterparts. Over 20 years of scientific research proved that a diet high in animal-based protein and fat, and low in dietary fiber and plant material increased the risk of Type 2 diabetes, vascular disease and cancer in the urban Chinese.[6]

In an era when the advances of medicine are venerated, it's hard to believe the best thing you can do for your health has nothing to do with technology. Research by prominent physicians Paul Ridker, M.D., K. Lance Gould, M.D., Peter Libby, M.D., and Dean Ornish, M.D., proved that the more you reduce vascular inflammation through comprehensive lifestyle changes, including an anti-inflammatory diet, regular exercise and stress reduction, the more you can diminish and even dry out the accumulation of plaque.[7]

In a landmark study published in the *Lancet*, Dr. Ornish put a group of heart patients on a low-fat, vegan diet with no dairy products and no meat. His patients were also told to exercise and meditate to better cope with stress. Within a year, the plaques in their coronary arteries had started to melt away, their chest pain ceased, and they were able to avoid going under the knife for bypass surgery or angioplasty.[8] His research proved that targeted "self-care" can reverse vascular disease. Another pioneer, Caldwell Esselstyn, Jr., M.D., had similar results when prescribing a low-fat, vegetarian diet to critically-ill heart patients at the Cleveland Clinic:

Just about everything had been tried—repeated open heart surgery, angioplasties, stents and a plethora of medications. Almost all the men were impotent, most had angina and, for some, things were so bad that they couldn't lie down and had to sleep sitting up. Of the patients who stuck to the program, there was not a single cardiac event over the next 12 years! All were alive and well and had reversed their disease.[9]

Vascular disease is a multi-factorial illness requiring a multi-factorial approach. The best way to treat the disease is to control what causes the disease to fester in the first place: inflammation. Research supports the use of very low-fat, vegetarian diets for controlling LDL cholesterol, slowing disease progression and reversing coronary artery disease. Higher-fat diets have been unsuccessful. Although low-fat, plant-based diets have been used with great success by some physicians and patients, they are not routinely encouraged by doctors.

Diet is given focus in this book because our country is in a SAD crisis of diet-related conditions: obesity, metabolic syndrome, Type 2 diabetes, hypertension, arthritis, certain cancers, depression and vascular disease. The overall increase in the weight of Americans, and the accompanying increase in the prevalence of diabetes, foreshadow a future with much higher rates of vascular disease.

American culture is a strange paradox. We have the highest rate of obesity on the planet, yet each year we spend about $40 billion on weight-loss programs, supplements and drugs. Evidence that dieting fails exists all around us. Although the rate of people who are moderately overweight has held steady over the past few decades, obesity has increased sharply, surpassing smoking as a major cause of death and disability. Today one-third of Americans—72 million—are at least 100 pounds over their ideal weight.

A Lifetime of Health Problems Ahead

One of the most disturbing trends in our country is the growing number of children who are obese. According to the CDC, childhood obesity has tripled since the mid 70s.[10] If you would sit outside a heart catheterization lab in any major hospital center, you would see a depressing number of really big kids in adult-size hospital gowns, waiting for a cardiovascular workup.

Obesity has made Type 2 diabetes more common among children and teenagers. Over 90 percent of new cases of diabetes in children occur in those who are obese. This dramatically increases their odds for cognitive decline, premature vascular disease and an early death. Antonio Convit, M.D., of the NYU School of Medicine, discovered that diabetes affects the brain's hippocampus, hampering attention, memory and other key aspects of cognition. He believes the toll is especially great on children, who may be impaired for life. One of the worst cases of an overweight child with Type 2 diabetes arrived in the hospital emergency room on a hot summer night when I was on call.

Fourteen-year-old Peter, whose name has been change to protect his identity, weighed over 300 pounds and was considered morbidly obese for his height. Earlier that day, Peter had dove into a four-foot deep pool and broke his neck, severing his spinal cord. He could no longer move his arms or his legs and would need a ventilator to breath. At an age when most teenage boys are experiencing an eruption of new feelings and sensations, Peter had lost all sensation in his young body. Worst of all, because of his enormous weight he wasn't a candidate for rehabilitation, unlike many quadriplegics who regain some functionality through hard work and physical therapy. The scientist and mathematician, Stephen Hawkings and journalist Charles Krauthammer, are two extraordinary examples of quadriplegics who have overcome their disabilities.

It would take 5-10 nurses and therapists to lift Peter's limp 300-pound-body out of bed and into a wheelchair. A special wheelchair would have to be made to accommodate his weight and paralysis. Until then, he would have to stay in his bed, which would have to be turned up-side-down at regular intervals to prevent his skin from breaking down, a complication of paralysis. The life ahead of Peter was full of unprecedented challenges in my field and the field of rehabilitation and medicine.

Many parents of obese children refuse to believe that their child is obese. They deny the consequences of their child's life-threatening condition. Nutritionist Ellyn Satter, a pioneer in the field of child feeding, says that parents are responsible for providing nutritious snacks and meals at regular intervals, and children are responsible for deciding whether they are hungry and how much to eat. But the child's caregiver holds the most power and responsibility for the nutritional life of their child. Today a quarter of a million children carry the Type 2 diagnosis.[11]

Obesity increases the risk of many cancers and illnesses, including metabolic syndrome, diabetes, renal and vascular disease, cancer, sexual dysfunction, arthritis and depression.

Fat and Inflammation

Fat, especially the visceral kind deep in the abdomen, generates bioactive substances that promote insulin resistance and inflammation. This affects every cell in the body, but especially the sensitive endothelial cells that line the walls of arteries. Specifically, visceral fat cells produce inflammatory cytokines, which trigger inflammation and the production of high levels of CRP. Silent, long-term inflammation can cause even more damage to the artery's endothelium than plaque.

Fat was necessary for survival because during the course of history, there was never a long period of uninterrupted food abundance. Famines were regular and frequent. Therefore, fat accumulation, when food was available, meant survival at times of shortage. Today scientists are comparing the belly fat to an organ, a gland or a tumor because of its intense metabolic activity. In a research study led by doctors at Harvard Medical School and Brigham and Women's Hospital, women with waists larger than 35 inches were 79 percent more likely to die prematurely than those with waists less than 27 inches, even if their weight was normal.[12] Visceral fat—that tire around your midsection—is often the first to go when you lose weight, which can reduce the odds of an early death.

Visceral fat also secretes a powerful hormone called leptin which communicates with the hypothalamus, the metabolic center of our brain. When fat stores are sufficient, leptin signals the brain to moderate our metabolism so that we don't gain weight. When we lose weight, fat cells shrink and leptin levels drop, signaling the brain to slow metabolism and conserve energy in fat stores. Genetic deficiencies in leptin can cause complex imbalances in metabolism that promote morbid obesity. But dieting is by far the number one cause of leptin imbalances that make losing weight difficult, a topic we discuss in Chapter 12.

Brain chemistry, yo-yo dieting, genetic mutations, addiction, culture and societal pressures are partly to blame for the American obesity epidemic. Some critics blame obesity on our easy access to cheap, processed "edible food things" that have replaced many of the nutrient-dense foods we routinely ate in the past. For millions of years, our ancestors ate a vegetarian diet of fresh fruits, vegetables and whole grains. Nor have we adapted to a food-chain disrupted by industrial by-products, pesticides and pollutants. But the surge in sugar, salt, animal protein and fat are by far generating the most damage in our bodies.

America's main course—meat—has more saturated fat and fewer nutrients, especially inflammation-fighting omega-3s, than a few decades ago, due to cost-saving changes to cattle feed. Saturated fat increases artery-clogging LDL-cholesterol. Unsaturated fats from complex carbohydrates like vegetables, fruit, legumes and whole grains lower the "bad" cholesterol. Saturated fat is also much harder to burn off. We only metabolize 3 percent of the fat we eat, the rest ends up in fat-stores in your belly, buttock or hips.

Most experts agree that Americans have gotten fatter and sicker because we've upset the balance of food intake, expenditure and storage (fat). In other words, we consume more calories than we burn off. The recommended daily caloric intake for healthy adults is 1,500-2,400 calories. Americans consume an average 4,200 calories per day. Many studies show that calorie restriction makes us live longer, and reduces the risk of cancer and vascular disease.

Americans also tend to eat the majority of their meals in restaurants, where dinner plates and portions have grown six to eight times larger in the past two decades. The house specialty at America's favorite steakhouse—the combination of a 20-ounce porterhouse steak, New York strip and large filet—exceeds the U.S. Department of Agriculture's (USDA) recommended daily meat intake by a whopping 15 ounces. A 20-ounce porterhouse steak provides about 1,750-2,000 calories—80 percent of them fat calories, and easily a day's worth of calories. And that's not including the large filet and New York Strip.

A century ago vascular disease was non-existent. Heart attacks and strokes were unheard of. By the middle of the century, vascular disease had become the leading cause of mortality. Alarmed by the growing rate of heart attacks and strokes, the U.S. Senate Select Committee on Nutrition held hearings in 1977 to investigate why. The committee discovered that while rates of vascular disease had soared in America since World War II, other cultures that had consumed a plant-based diet had much lower rates of the disease. Epidemiologists who testified also observed that during the rationing of dairy and meat in World War II, the rate of vascular disease had declined in our country.

As a result of the government's findings, the committee crafted a new set of U.S. dietary guidelines, calling on Americans to cut down on red meat and dairy products:

> Within weeks a firestorm, emanating from the red-meat and dairy industries, engulfed the committee, and Senator McGovern (who had a great many cattle ranchers among his South Dakota constituents) was forced to beat a retreat ... "Reduce consumption of meat" was replaced by artful compromise: "Choose meats, poultry and fish that will reduce saturated-fat intake."[13]

Michael Pollan noted that when it comes to the food industry, decisions are often driven by politics and economics—not science, not common sense, and certainly not the health of Americans.

The secret to losing weight and stopping, or reversing vascular disease is in the whole foods aisle. Inflammation-fighting antioxidants in fruits and vegetables can be identified by their rich, vibrant colors—the bright orange of carrots; the deep red of tomatoes; the yellow of squash and corn; and the dark-purple of blueberries, blackberries and grapes. Fruits and vegetables also give our circulatory system the vital nutrients that allow it to function effectively. About 80 percent of the foods you eat should be unrefined plant foods. Regression of vascular disease has been proved by coronary angiography and cardiac positron emission tomography (PET) scans, only with this type of diet.

Studies show that if your weight, cholesterol, blood pressure and blood glucose are kept under control, your risk of developing vascular disease is only five percent. But the reality is that most U.S. adults with diabetes or high blood pressure don't have it under control. This makes them vulnerable to heart attacks, strokes, disability, dementia, kidney and heart failure, and ultimately, a diminished quality of life. Experts claim that the rising obesity rates in children may mean the next generation will have a shorter life span than their parents. For adults and children at risk, or who already have a diet-related disease or condition, changing eating habits is a small price to pay for a longer life. In the following chapters, we'll explore how the age-old secrets of No-Dieting can help you lose weight and achieve optimal health.

PART I:
THE NO-DIETING SECRETS

CHAPTER 1

STARCHY FOODS: NATURE'S FAT BURNERS

Our bodies need two broad categories of chemicals on a regular basis: macronutrients, substances that we need to consume in larger quantities, and micronutrients, substances that we need in small amounts. Three major classes of macronutrients are essential to our health and well-being: carbohydrates, fats and proteins.

The low-carbohydrate craze and ensuing widespread carbophobia changed the way Americans look at the most fat-burning, satiating and nutrient-dense food group, carbohydrates. Starchy carbohydrates, like potatoes, corn, peas, whole-wheat pasta, multi-grain bread, kasha and brown rice (plus many other whole grains, fruits, legumes and vegetables), are the same food group that our ancestors ate for thousands and thousands of years. Common sense and modern medical science beg us to rethink our aversion to carbohydrates, but many Americans continue to tell themselves that eating a 12-ounce slab of prime rib is healthier than eating a baked potato. Carbohydrates are the body's first choice for fuel, and the only nutrient that can effectively get to the brain and nervous system. They are nature's fat burners.

The commercial genius of the high-protein, low-carbohydrate diet was that Americans were told they can maintain their love of cheeseburgers, steak, bacon and eggs and still lose weight. It was a devilish deal for the price of later complications such as hypertension, stroke, and clogged coronary arteries. Another reason why low-carbohydrate diets are popular, despite all the long-term health costs, is that they fit the American conspiracy mindset. Who wouldn't like to believe that thousands of scientific studies correlating the consumption of meat and dairy products with chronic disease were a big, fat lie?

Complex vs. Simple Carbohydrates

Carbohydrates are not all the same. The *amount* of carbohydrates in our diet doesn't affect us as much as the *quality* of those carbohydrates because our bodies metabolize *simple* and *complex* carbohydrates at different rates. Processing robs complex carbohydrates of key nutrients and fat-burning starch, and turns them into simple carbohydrates, short chains of sugar molecules. Complex carbohydrates in fresh foods such as cantaloupes, lentils and winter squash are made of long chains of sugar molecules and starch. These will line the digestive track and bind with water and cholesterol, leaving you full for much longer periods of time and even removing cholesterol from your bloodstream. High-fat, high-caloric protein foods like chicken, beef or cheese add cholesterol.

The best news is that we lose about 25 percent of the calories from Brussels sprouts, broccoli, Navy beans, oranges and other complex carbohydrates in the energy spent while metabolizing. We lose only 10 percent of the calories from simple carbohydrates while metabolizing. The other 90 percent will end-up as stored fat on our hips and bellies. Green and yellow vegetables, oatmeal, black beans and other complex carbohydrates increase the thermic effect of food (TEF). They turn up our internal furnace, burning calories as heat and energy rather than converting them into fat. Even if we eat an excessive amount of carbohydrates, we will burn more calories in the energy spent converting them into glycogen, a high-octane reserve fuel stored in our liver, kidneys and muscles.

Another huge benefit of the bulky fiber and starch in vegetables, whole grains, legumes and fruits is that they take more energy to digest and break down into the bloodstream, prolonging the digestive process and increasing our resting metabolic rate (RMR). The energy expended at rest, our RMR, supports the work of our vital organs, such as the brain, heart and lungs. A faster RMR means that more calories will be burned at rest—the easy way to lose weight.

At the molecular level, carbohydrates, fats and protein have varying effects on our bodies. The conversion of complex carbohydrates to fat cells is a rare event. Even if we overeat nature's fat burners, we'll still lose 25 percent of the calories in the energy spent while metabolizing, and another 20 percent of the calories converting them to glycogen. But, eating calories from simple carbohydrates versus complex carbohydrate calories will make you eat more calories.

SECRET: All carbohydrates are not alike. *Starchy* complex carbohydrates satiate hunger and turn up our internal furnace, burning calories as heat and energy. High-sugar, high-fat *simple* carbohydrates increase hunger, addiction and cravings.

Western Diseases

The second big advantage of starchy foods was discovered by the "Father of the Fiber Revolution," Dennis Burkitt, M.D., who correlated Western diseases with our modern SAD diet of increased amounts of meat, processed foods, and fewer fruits, whole grains and vegetables. These diseases include obesity, diabetes, vascular disease and cancer. The Asians and Africans Dr. Burkitt studied ate a more traditional fiber-rich diet of cassava, yams, millet, beans, whole grain rice, starchy fruits and green vegetables, and enjoyed much lower rates of Western diseases.

In Dr. Campbell's China Study, whole foods rich in starch made up 90 percent of the traditional diet eaten by the disease-free Chinese in traditional villages. Their average cholesterol level was only 127 mg/dl, close to 100 points below the American average of 215 mg/dl.[14] Root vegetables such as carrots and rutabaga, whole-grain rice and unprocessed cereals such as corn, barley and oats are some of the most fiber-rich carbohydrates.

Late nineteenth-century inventions in wheat farming and flour milling marked a turning point in the American diet, forever changing our basic food staples such as bread products. Revolutionary steel and porcelain grinders in flour mills began to convert wheat, corn and other grains into superfine flour, eliminating two of the most nutrient-dense components of whole grains. The grinding removed the germ and the bran (the outer husk) from the wheat kernel, and then crushed the inner kernel into flour. Flour mills were an important part of rural communities across the country.

SECRET: The same starchy carbohydrates that promote weight loss can prevent, *stop* and even *reverse* disease

Fiber controls the rate of digestion and has complex physiological effects on the digestive system and brain. It offers a variety of benefits such as lowering cholesterol, absorbing fat and reducing the risk of colon cancer. Fiber is the only dietary factor that has convincing evidence showing a protective effect against weight gain and obesity.[15]

As fiber passes through the digestive tract it absorbs minerals and eliminates fat, cholesterol and cancer-causing toxins. Up to a third of fibrous, starchy, complex carbohydrates are excreted by your body as waste. They *resist* digestion and provide few calories. Most simple carbohydrates like cake, cookies and white bread are broken down into sugars that your body rapidly absorbs and stores as fat. When "resistant starch" reaches the small intestine, bacteria use it as fuel, a process called fermentation that protects colon cells from cancer. The starch travels undigested all the way through the small intestine. You literally *waste* more of the calories from starchy complex carbohydrates. Another benefit is that fiber and resistant starch help promote insulin sensitivity.

SECRET: The "resistant starch" in complex carbohydrates absorbs fat and cholesterol, and defies digestion while providing few calories and the feeling of fullness.

The new refined flour could last longer and pack a better taste punch: as soon as the flour mixes with our saliva, it turns into sugar and raises insulin levels. A higher level of insulin in your blood means that your body will burn more blood sugar, giving you a nice jolt of energy but little else. Cells burn sugars preferentially. In an hour or so after the Wonder Bread is gone, not only will your energy level plummet, your gut and brain will stimulate your appetite again. And off to the refrigerator you'll go. Insulin is one of the key hormones involved in appetite. Our obesity epidemic is, in part, an epidemic of *hyper-insulinemia*. Even those diet soft drinks that we consume trick our bodies and brains into stimulating our appetite. To avoid feeling tired and hungry all the time, skip the soft drinks and simple carbs and choose foods that are rich in fiber, such as those listed in Figure 2.

Simple carbohydrates are found in most commercial white breads, white rice, pretzels, French fries, beer and all the varieties of potato chips, soft drinks, baked goods and candy bars. In our SAD diet, simple carbohydrates contribute about half of all calories and very few nutrients. Our bodies can break down simple carbohydratess quickly, resulting in an addicting but short-lived sugar high. The greater number of simple carbohydrates in your diet, the higher the "glycemic load" or spike in blood sugar will be. As sugar levels in the blood rise, so does insulin. Surges of insulin push the body to store the excess sugar as fat. Chronic surges in insulin lead to chronic inflammation, weight gain, Type 2 diabests and high cholesterol.[16] High-glycemic foods decrease the "good" HDL cholesterol that protects our arteries (see Figure: 1). In a recent study, children who ate a lot of sugary carbohydrates had much higher cholesterol levels.[17]

Figure 1: Correlation between glycemic load and HDL cholesterol.

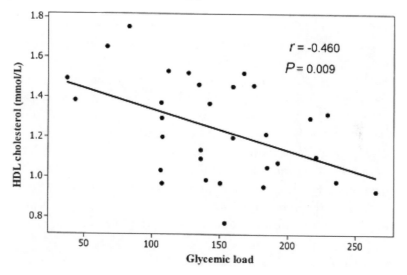

SECRET: Refined carbohydrates reduce the "good" HDL cholesterol and increase triglycerides, insulin levels, blood pressure and fat stores—all proven culprits in the development of inflammation and chronic disease.

Unlucky Charms

Hunger and satiety are not the only reasons we start and stop eating. Researchers in the burgeoning field of food psychology have pinpointed a complex web of cues in the modern environment that all but overwhelm our adaptive systems: colors, presentation, portions and food packaging. Parents can marvel at the multitude of cereal brands that promulgate the colorful, overcrowded cereal aisle. "Lucky Charms," the most popular children's breakfast cereal on the market, boasts "Whole Grains" on the front of the box. But the amount of simple-sugars found in one cup of the breakfast cereal cancels any

Great Grains
- Wheat
- Oatmeal
- Corn
- Popcorn
- Brown rice
- Whole rye
- Barley
- Bulgur
- Millet
- Buckwheat
- Quinoa
- Sorghum

nutritional value of the grains. Refined carbs offer a sweet taste and short-lived surge of energy that can be very addicting, especially for young children. Simple carbs are sugars. Limit your total consumption of sugar to 10 percent or less of your daily calories to prevent the effects of insulin resistance.

Refined grains, such as white flour and white rice, have been processed, which removes nutrients and fiber. Unrefined grains still contain these vitamins and minerals, and are rich in fiber, which helps your digestive system work well. Fiber also helps you feel full, so you're less likely to overeat. That explains why a bowl of oatmeal fills you up better than sugary cereal which has the same amount of calories as the oatmeal.

Best of all, whole grains help prevent vascular disease. In the Iowa Women's Health Study of 34,000 women, those who ate at least one serving of whole grains each day had a 30 to 40 percent lower risk of vascular disease than women who ate no whole grains.[18]

Be Wary of Breads with a Fake Tan

Consumers should be wary of deceptive advertising when it comes to whole grains. Manufacturers advertise many cereals, breads, crackers, pretzels and even pasta products as "Whole Grain," but in reality these products are primarily made of white flour, sugar, chemicals, and additives, including caramel coloring. Coarsely ground grains curtail our appetite better and provide disease-fighting nutrients. Check the label of ingredients to watch out for "Whole Grain" products with a fake tan. If multi-grains, wheat, corn, rice, bulgur, millet, oats or another grain aren't listed within the first two ingredients, move on to the next loaf.

Maximizing Nutrients

Freshness, preparation and cooking make a difference in maximizing the amount of nutrients you receive from unprocessed carbohydrates. Slightly green bananas have more resistant starch and less sugar than ripened bananas. If you cool cooked starches, such as potatoes and whole-wheat pasta, you can increase the amount of resistant starch in the food. Pasta should be cooked "al dente" (slightly firm).The more you cook pasta, the faster it is broken down into sugar. Cooking carrots releases more nutrients than if you would eat the vegetable raw. But overcooking vegetables can ruin a perfectly good source of disease-fighting nutrients. Overcooking vegetables reduces the amount of phytochemicals, vitamins and other nutrients that enter our body.

Many people think that complex carbohydrates such as potatoes are fattening. A big potato has almost no fat, no cholesterol and is high in fiber. But if you add butter and sour cream, you're transforming an ideal food into one very high in fat and cholesterol. The trick is to eat a small potato and dress it up without adding fats. If you consume 100 calories of fat, you'll lose only three percent of the calories while metabolizing. The rest, or 97 percent, of the fat calories will be hanging from your abdomen or hips by the next day or within the week.

Bountiful Beans

Legumes or beans contain a lot of resistant starch that we digest slowly or not at all. They also have a low glycemic load.

• Adzuki beans
• Black beans
• Black-eyed peas
• Butter beans
• Calico beans
• Cannellini beans
• Edamame
• Fava beans
• Garbanzo beans
• Great Northern beans
• Kidney beans
• Lentils
• Lima beans
• Mung beans
• Navy beans
• Pinto beans
• Soy beans
• Split Peas

Choose Foods that Burn Fat

Understanding and taking advantage of how your body uses and stores energy is the key to good health and maximum weight loss. Your cells metabolize energy, or calories, from protein, carbohydrates and fats. Calories "in" are not calories "out." It takes more calories to digest and metabolize the starch and nutrients in complex carbohydrates. It takes much less energy, or calories, to metabolize fats and simple sugars. Your body stores complex carbohydrates within cells as glycogen, a nutrient that the body can easily and rapidly convert to energy.

Foods that promote weight loss are high in complex carbohydrates. Your body requires much more energy to break down and digest their critical nutrients. When you eat high complex carbohydrate foods such as whole grains, fruits and vegetables, your body increases your metabolism, which in turn promotes weight loss. In fact, you'll lose 45 percent of the calories from complex carbohydrates during digestion alone. Often times these foods have fewer calories than it takes the body to process and use them. The increase in metabolism can burn excess body fat. Nutritious foods promote weight loss!

SECRET: Foods that promote weight loss are high in complex carbohydrates which take more energy (calories) to break down. Your metabolism speeds up to process the critical nutrients in these foods. A faster metabolism can burn excess body fat.

Complex Carbohydrates on the Brain

Food also affects our brain chemistry, for better or worse. Tryptophan is one of the essential amino acids that our brain uses to synthesize serotonin, a powerful neurotransmitter. Serotonin improves mood, reduces appetite and induces sleep, among other things. High-protein foods such as beef, turkey and fish contain high levels of tryptophan, but they also have large quantities of the other amino acids that compete with tryptophan to reach the brain. Protein actually has a negative effect on tryptophan and serotonin levels. Studies have shown that women on a high-protein diet tend to have trouble sleeping, this may be partially due to the reduction in serotonin.

According to research by Drs. Richard and Judith Wurtman of the Massachusetts Institute of Technology, insulin drives long-chained amino acids out of blood circulation and into tissues and organs. Eating lots of low-protein, high-carbohydrate starches, vegetables and fruits, raises insulin that encourages amino acids to leave blood circulation with the result that more tryptophan can enter the brain. When the

SECRET: Consumption of complex carbohydrates helps the brain produce higher levels of serotonin which reduces your appetite and increases your feeling of well-being.

supply of tryptophan increases, serotonin increases and appetite decreases. And that is one important reason why complex carbohydrates turn off the appetite and create a feeling of satisfaction.

Getting Over Carbophobia

When the trillion-dollar food industry throws its marketing weight behind a dieting fad, our perception of a certain type of food can change, for better or for worse. Americans have been conditioned to believe that all carbohydrates are bad, and they are starving for carbohydrates as a result. The Institute of Medicine, the unit of the National Academies that sets our recommended daily intake values for nutrients, has set 130 grams of carbohydrates as the recommended minimum daily intake for adults and children.

Animal-based products such as meat, dairy and eggs—the foods richest in artery-clogging cholesterol—are deficient in fiber. Beef, fish and poultry have no starch. Foods rich in protein also decrease serotonin levels. The sugar rush you crave after the average high protein, high fat American meal is your body's attempt to fill that hole of satisfaction. Complex carbohydrates also fuel our brains.

As we chew food, our saliva releases a digestive enzyme called alpha amylase that is crucial for breaking down starch into glucose. Our brains run on glucose. Primates and other animals with smaller brains lack the genetic code to manufacturer the enzyme. Evolutionary scientists theorize that our unique ability to digest starchy carrots, onions and potatoes gave our ancestors enough glucose to develop large brains over time. And when our body metabolizes starch, the resulting by-products,

High-fiber Foods
- Rhubarb
- Spinach
- Sprouts
- Raisins
- Prunes
- Peppers
- Cabbage
- Carrots
- Eggplant
- Kale
- Lettuce
- Corn
- Cauliflower
- Okra
- Onions
- Beets
- Broccoli
- Berries
- Apples
- Cranberries
- Dates
- Figs
- Grapes
- Mangoes

carbon dioxide and water are easily eliminated from the body. In contrast, animal protein requires much more effort to convert into energy, and its by-product, nitrogen, converts to ammonia and urea, both of which can be harmful to the vascular system, kidneys and liver. The bottom line is that our body handles starchy carbohydrates more efficiently, leaving us more feeling more alert, energized and satisfied.

Starch: Nature's Statin

Starchy complex carbohydrates, vegetables, legumes, whole grains and fruit offer fiber, antioxidants and minerals. Fiber blocks synthesis of cholesterol, slows down glucose absorption and controls the rate of digestion. Many carbohydrates even resist digestion. They're our best weapon against the trio of insulin resistance, obesity and vascular disease.

The simple carbohydrates in white pasta, white bread and other refined foods are not only stripped of disease-fighting nutrients and fiber, they stimulate our pancreas to produce insulin. If we eat too many simple carbohydrates, our body begins to store the excess glucose as fat. Overindulging on simple carbohydrates can lead to insulin resistance and obesity.

For the health conscious eater, complex carbohydrates offer several major benefits: they take longer to digest and some of their calories are eliminated; they keep water in the gut, promoting satiety; and they reduce cholesterol. Best of all, unprocessed carbohydrates improve our mood and provide sustained energy. The strongest evidence for a way of eating that prolongs lifespan is for starchy, complex carbohydrates—nature's miracle fat-burners and nutritional winners.

Fat-burning, High-fiber, Nutritional Knock-outs

Asparagus	Black Beans	Oranges	Peppers
Broccoli	Turnip Greens	Pinto Beans	Cherries
Brussels sprouts	Winter Squash	Pumpernickel	Blueberries
Sprouts	Buckwheat	Cauliflower	Garbanzo Beans
Cabbage	Kale	Multi-grain	Prunes
Carrots	Brown Rice	Prunes	Pineapple
Celery	Whole-wheat Pasta	Pineapple	Apples
Corn	Kasha	Grapefruit	Mango
Cucumbers	Couscous	Figs	Apples
Eggplant	Millet	Grapes	Boysenberries
Lettuce	Bulgur	Kiwi Fruit	Bananas (slightly green)
Navy Beans	Lentils	Cranberries	Sorghum
Okra	Pearled Barley	Nectarines	Pears
Onions	Oatmeal	Mushrooms	Raspberries
Peas	Wheatabix Cereal	Papaya	Melon
Potatoes	Bran Cereal	Peaches	Blueberries
Spinach	Blackberries	Pineapple	Cantaloupe
Tomatoes	Kidney Beans	Rhubarb	Strawberries
Water cress	All-Bran	Watermelon	Walnuts
Zucchini	Prunes	Radishes	Multi-grain bread
Yams	Quinoa	Cassava	Squash
Flax seed	Collard greens	Endive	Romaine lettuce
Chicory	Millet	Triticale	Buckwheat
Barley	Popcorn	Rye	Chard

Figure 2: A list of fat-burning, high-fiber, nutritional knock-outs.

CHAPTER 2
FATS: THE GOOD, THE BAD AND THE TERRIBLE

Jack, a 73 year old patient with severe vascular disease, found himself at the side of the road in a ditch after a mini-stroke, a trans ischemic attack or TIA. One of his carotid arteries, that supplies oxygen and nutrients to his brain, was blocked. He had been told by his cardiologist to "get his affairs together," and that if he did not have a stent to open the blockage, within the month he would be dead from either a massive stroke or heart attack. Jack was on seven different medications. His first stent opened a blocked artery in his heart. The procedure was such a miserable experience he said he would rather just die than have to go through a second stenting. His cardiologist referred him to me, hoping that I might be able to help.

I first saw Jack about six years ago. Today he plays tennis three times a week and plays golf on the weekend. Jack and his wife help their daughter with her two young children two days a week by babysitting, allowing his daughter to work part time. He takes no medications whatsoever, and has not needed any additional medical procedures or surgery. Jack followed the secrets of the Non Diet, choosing a low-fat, near-vegetarian way of eating. Dr. Dean Ornish and others proved that such changes reverse vascular disease, decrease angina, bring about permanent weight loss, and reduce premature deaths from fatal arrhythmias, stroke and heart attack. If you are going to reverse disease, you need to get to the root of the disease. And the root is always going to be at the molecular or cellular level.

Is the Real Enemy Fat?

For almost 30 years, scientists, physicians, nutritionists and journalists lambasted dietary fat. This spawned a billion-dollar *low-fat* and *fat-free* food market with margarine leading the list as the less tasty, but supposedly healthier, replacement for butter. Decades later, scientists "discovered" that the trans fat in margarine was worse for your health than the saturated fat in butter.

All fat is not bad. The greater the number of hydrogen atoms in fat, the denser or more *saturated* the fat is, and the worse it will be for your health. Today, nutritionists and physicians differentiate between the "bad" saturated and "terrible" trans-fatty acids, found in animal products and processed foods, and the "good" unsaturated fats found mainly in fish, nuts, seeds and plant oils. During the low-fat craze, Americans cut these critically important fats.

Dietary fat is an essential nutrient and energy source for organs and muscles. Your body needs it to produce cell membranes, as well as eicosanoids, hormone-like messengers that help control inflammation and blood clotting. Fat also helps absorb vitamins that promote healthy skin, hair and nails. Your nervous system needs fat to function properly, the brain relies on it to cushion and protect the membranes of brain cells (neurons). About 60 percent of the human brain is fat.[19]

Dietary fat has more than twice the energy (calories) of carbohydrates or protein. All types of fat are easily converted to fat and stored in your body for future use. Only three percent of the calories from fat are lost in metabolism for things like cellular growth and repair. The rest, or 97 percent, of their calories will be stored in your abdomen, buttocks or hips. Protein and complex carbohydrates are metabolized more efficiently and are less likely to be converted to fat. But a low-fat label is not a license to eat a bigger portion. Many fat-free foods are loaded with sugar, corn syrup and calories. You should treat them as carefully as you would full-fat products that you wouldn't eat in excess.

SECRET: Reducing saturated fat without reducing refined carbohydrates works against the goal to lose weight and prevent or reverse chronic disease.

Dietary Fat and Disease

Heavy consumption of saturated fats can cause inflammation and lead to changes in your body that make blood clot more easily, increasing your risk of a heart attack or stroke. And whole and 2 percent milk, cheese, cream, veal, beef, pork, lamb are high in saturated fat.

Monounsaturated, and especially polyunsaturated, fats appear to reduce inflammation and LDL oxidation within the arteries.[20] These fats clean out artery-clogging LDL cholesterol, strengthening your heart and vascular system. Plant-based fats are as essential to human nutrition as vitamins and minerals. Polyunsaturated fats are divided into omega-3 and omega-6 fatty acids.

The omegas are called essential fatty acids. We need to get these from food, our bodies cannot make them. Essential fatty acids regulate the balance of saturated fat and cholesterol in cells. Without the omegas, infants would develop heart, brain and liver disorders. Children would experience growth retardation, impaired vision and emotional disorders.

The omega-3 fatty acids derived from the fats in walnuts, flaxseeds, some fruits and vegetables, and fish haven't been hydrogenated, and do not appear to have the same corrosive effect on our arteries as saturated and trans fats. Omega-3s also improve insulin sensitivity and suppress inflammation in the bloodstream, joints and tissues.

Lower Dietary Cholesterol
- Increase consumption of fruits, vegetables, beans and whole grains
- Choose margarines that are low in satarated fats, and cooking oils that are high in unsaturated fats such as olive, corn, and canola oils. Avoid saturated and trans fats.
- Eliminate meats and consume little or no dairy products, including eggs, cheese and butter.

Salmon is very good to eat because of the omega-3 acids. A comprehensive review of nearly 100 studies exploring different diets and cholesterol-lowering agents showed just how beneficial the omega-3 fatty acids in fish can be to our hearts. In studies of people who consume diets rich in omega-3 fatty acids, the risks of vascular disease, stroke and heart attack was 23 percent lower compared to a control group.[21] Sardines, anchovies and herring also have high levels of omega-3s. Sardines may not seem like a health food, but they are high in omega-3s and contain virtually no mercury. They also have lots of calcium and other critical vitamins and minerals.

Safflower, cottonseed and soybean oils are common sources of omega-6 fatty acids. The omega-6s help lower cholesterol, fight infections and improve blood viscosity so our blood is able to clot. But when omega-6s aren't balanced with sufficient amounts of omega-3s, problems ensue. Our SAD diet averages 20-30 times more omega-6s than omega-3s. And while omega-6s may lower cholesterol, omega-3s can actually clean out the plaque in arteries.

Americans consume far too much omega-6s, found in most polyunsaturated vegetable oils, and not enough of omega-3s. Omega-3s are found in fish, fish oils, eggs from properly fed chickens, dark-green vegetables and herbs, oils from certain seeds such as flax and chia, nuts such as walnuts, and in small amounts in all whole grains.[22]

Three decades of low-fat dieting left many Americans with a deficiency in omega-3s, contributing to the epidemics of asthma, arthritis, cancer, depression and vascular disease. These diseases are a type of inflammation. If you eat a diet deficient in the "good" fats and abundant in the "bad" fats, or one that is high in sugar, fructose or corn syrup, you are increasing the rate of inflammation in your body and getting down to the roots of chronic disease.

SECRET: Saturated fats increase artery-clogging LDL-cholesterol. The unsaturated fats in oily fish, walnuts, flaxseeds, and plant-based oils reduce LDL-cholesterol, inflammation and plaque within blood vessels.

Investigations of the Greenland Eskimo diet and disease patterns led to important discoveries on the role of the omegas and inflammation. Scientists discovered that our bodies produce inflammatory messengers from converting omega-6s into fatty arachidonic acid (AA). An overabundance of inflammatory messengers plays a major role in chronic disease. When you increase your consumption of nutritious whole foods, you'll produce fewer of the messengers that cause inflammation and disease.

The Terrible Trans Fats

Saturated, trans fat has twice the potential to damage your heart in comparison to the fat found in meat and dairy products. Greasy french fries, donuts, potato chips and pastries, foods high in trans fatty acids, raise artery-clogging LDL-cholesterol more than any other dietary factor.

As an engineered food additive, trans fat improves the stability and longevity of processed foods. It doesn't spoil as easily as non-hydrogenated fat. But as a dietary factor, trans fat is terrible. Biochemists, physicians and nutritionists now know that trans fat promotes disease through *multiple* biochemical mechanisms.

Trans fat *raises* the "bad" LDL-cholesterol and triglycerides, the smaller, more dense particles which may damage the arteries. If that isn't bad enough, trans fat also lowers the "good" HDL-cholesterol which cleans out blood vessels. Even consuming low levels of trans fat, one to two percent of your daily calories, increases your risk of vascular disease by 25 percent.[23]

Trans Fatty Foods
- Biscuits
- Breakfast bars (some)
- Cookies
- Crackers
- Cream
- Doughnuts
- Fried foods (some)
- Pastries
- Lard (shortening)
- Margarine
- Salad Dressing (some)
- Potato Chips

The food industry produces trans fat by adding hydrogen to vegetable oil, a process called "hydrogenation." Lard, a common ingredient in baked goods and fried foods often contains high levels of trans fat. Trans fat has *zero* nutritional value and lots and lots of calories. One gram of trans fat is 10 calories, one gram of protein or carbohydrates is only four calories.

Avoiding the fat takes some effort, since deep-fried fast food is full of it, although that may be changing. McDonald's announced in May 2008 that their fries will no longer be cooked in trans fatty lard. Smaller, less commercial restaurants don't have the same pressure to eliminate trans fat and may still use it in rolls, desserts and fried foods.

"We estimate that if we replaced all the trans fats in the American diet with polyunsaturated fats from vegetable sources, we could reduce the national risk of type 2 diabetes by up to 40 percent," said Dr. Walter Willett, a nutritional epidemiologist at Harvard University.[24] Researchers at Harvard calculated that eliminating the fat from the U.S. food supply could prevent up to 20 percent of heart attacks and related deaths each year.[25] To be on the safe side, look for products, including frozen breakfast foods, margarine and vegetable oils which contain no trans fats. All commercially-packaged food products must list any trans

SECRET: Trans fat offers what the Mayo Clinic calls "the cholesterol double-whammy," it raises "bad" LDL-cholesterol and lowers "good" HDL-cholesterol. The greater the percentage of trans fat in a food product, the higher risk is for heart attack and stroke.

fat content on their nutrition labe. But marketing claims of "trans fat-free" do not address the amount of artery-clogging *saturated* fat in the food item.

From Your Lips to Your Hips

Plant-based oils are rich in heart-healthy unsaturated fats but *use oils sparingly*. Some, such as coconut and palm oil, contain more saturated fats than animal products. Ounce for ounce, olive oil is one of the most fattening, caloric-dense foods on the planet. It packs even more calories per pound than butter, which averages 3,000 calories a pound. Olive oil has, on average, 4,000 calories per pound—at least *twice* the calories of white sugar. It's also more easily stored as fat than sugar.

Your body requires very little energy to process oils which means most of the calories will be stored as fat. Your body deposits fat in the abdomen (omentum) and the subcutaneous fat between your skin and muscles. Fat may also be deposited in your blood vessels where it can block blood flow and damage organs.[26]

SECRET: Try to eliminate olive and other cooking oils while trying to lose weight, and then use them sparingly. Fish or a teaspoon of ground flaxseeds or walnuts offers the benefits of omega-3 fatty acids without all the fat of oil.

Your body stores over 40 billion fat cells in the tissue thread between your skin, organs and muscle walls. Fat cells are like balloons filled with greasy lipids. When you lose weight the "balloons" deflate. If you consume more fat calories than you burn off, the "balloons" inflate. Too much inflation can become toxic.

Excess fat in the omentum, an organ in your belly that sends hormone-like messages to your immune system and brain, generates inflammatory substances that contribute to disease, disability and premature death. In one of the largest, longest health studies in the world, researchers found that belly fat *doubled* death risk. Premature death increased with waist circumference: the wider the waist, the greater the risk.[27]

When calculating the recommended daily allowance (RDA) of macronutrients (protein, carbohydrates, and fat), the USDA recommends that adults consume 20-35 percent, and children consume up to 40 percent of their calories from dietary fat. Past RDAs kept fat fewer than 30 percent. But for people with several risk factors for vascular disease, or for those who have the disease, even 30 percent is too high. We recommend 25 percent. The USDA also does not differentiate between "good" fats and "bad" fats, despite mounting evidence correlating saturated fat with obesity and disease, and vegetable-based fats with much lower rates of disease.[28]

If you're trying to lose weight or reverse disease, use heart-healthy cooking oils sparingly, replace whole or 2 percent dairy products with low-fat ones, and eat more starchy foods. The fiber in fruits, vegetables and whole grains helps block the absorption of fat and fills you up, you won't feel deprived and will gain energy and stamina, not weight.

Diet-related Cancers
- Bladder cancer
- Brain cancer
- Breast cancer
- Colon cancer
- Endometrial cancer
- Intestinal cancer
- Kidney cancer
- Leukemia
- Lung cancer
- Lymphoma
- Mouth cancer
- Ovarian cancer
- Pancreatic cancer
- Prostate cancer
- Skin cancer
- Stomach cancer

Fats to Avoid	
Saturated Fats: Butter, cheese, whole milk and ice-cream; meat; snack foods; chocolate bars; coconut and palm oils	Saturated fats raise total blood cholesterol as well as "bad" LDL cholesterol.
Trans Fats: Partially-hydrogenated vegetable oil; French fries; baked goods; margarine	Trans fats raise LDL cholesterol and lower "good" HDL cholesterol.
Fats to Use Sparingly	
Monounsaturated Fats: Olive, peanut, rapeseed, and canola oils; peanut butter; avocados; cashews, walnuts and almonds	Monounsaturated fats lower total cholesterol and LDL cholesterol and increase the HDL cholesterol.
Polyunsaturated Fats: Soybean, safflower, corn, and cottonseed oils; walnuts; fatty fish	Polyunsaturated fats also lower total cholesterol and LDL cholesterol. Omega-3 fatty acids belong to this group and have the unique quality of reversing plaque.

Figure 3: A guide to the different types of dietary fat.

Percentage of Specific Types of Fat in Common Oils and Fats*

Oils	Saturated	Monounsaturated	Polyunsaturated	Trans
Canola	7	58	29	0
Safflower	9	12	74	0
Sunflower	10	20	66	0
Corn	13	24	60	0
Olive	13	72	8	0
Soybean	16	44	37	0
Peanut	17	49	32	0
Palm	50	37	10	0
Coconut	87	6	2	0
Cooking Fats				
Shortening	22	29	29	18
Lard	39	44	11	1
Butter	60	26	5	5
Margarine/Spreads				
70% Soybean Oil, Stick	18	2	29	23
67% Corn & Soybean Oil Spread, Tub	16	27	44	11
48% Soybean Oil Spread, Tub	17	24	49	8
60% Sunflower, Soybean, and Canola Oil Spread, Tub	18	22	54	5

Values expressed as percent of total fat; data are from analyses at Harvard School of Public Health Lipid Laboratory and U.S.D.A. publications.

CHAPTER 3
PROTEIN: RETHINKING MEAT

Our circulatory, metabolic and digestive systems have not changed in any substantial way in millions of years, but our way of agriculture and eating has radically changed. Before the epidemic of Type 2 diabetes, obesity and vascular disease, two-thirds of our protein came from plant foods. Cattle roamed the prairies and grazed on grass, which is a good source of omega-3s. Like cattle, chickens are now kept in cramped pens and sometimes even force-fed. Americans eat, on average, 87 pounds of chicken and 66 pounds of beef per person per year—a whopping 314 percent increase in chicken and 50 percent increase in beef consumption over the past century. Our consumption rate of meat is roughly twice the global average.[29]

Dean Ornish, M.D. once said, "I don't understand why asking people to eat a well-balanced vegetarian diet is considered drastic, while it is medically conservative to cut people open." Several studies correlating the cholesterol and saturated fat in red meat with inflammation convinced American consumers to eat less red meat and more fish and poultry. This actually increased our total consumption of animal protein as we got better at factory-style chicken and fish farming. We consume about 50 percent more animal protein than our recommended daily allowance. Our consumption of fruits and vegetables falls short of recommended levels. Contrary to popular belief, we can get all the protein our bodies need from plants. A hundred calories of Romaine lettuce has twice the protein of 100 calories of beef. And plant-based protein is much healthier because it has lots of fiber and nutrients, no fat and virtually no cholesterol.

How Much Protein Do We Need?

Digestion of animal protein begins in the stomach where acids and enzymes begin to break it down into smaller components called amino acids. Many of our bodies' most important chemicals—enzymes,

SECRET: Animal protein raises cholesterol while plant protein lowers it. Meat also raises artery-clogging saturated fat.

hormones, neurotransmitters and even our DNA are at least partially comprised of protein. Our bodies also use protein to build muscles and tissues, but athletes and body builders know that the maximum muscle mass they can build in a week is one pound. Excess protein is excreted by our kidneys and liver and is hard on the vascular system. Although our bodies can "recycle" protein, we use it up constantly, so we must continually replace it.

The amount of protein you need each day is a function of your lean body mass, not your body weight if you are overweight. The Institute of Medicine set the recommended daily allowance for protein at about 7 grams per 20 pounds. These figures vary widely but most of us would do just fine on 30 grams of protein a day, virtually *all* of it from plant sources. Combining legumes, such as lentils, with green leafy vegetables is the best strategy to make sure you get the protein you need. Complex carbohydrate vegetables, fruits, whole grains and legumes contain more than 50 grams of protein per 1,000 calories. If you eat a healthy balance of these foods every day, you'll consume more than enough protein to meet your daily metabolic needs.

> **SECRET:** To get the minimum amount of protein you need each day, balance your vegetables with beans and, if you're not on a diet, nuts.

Animal Protein and Disease

Animal protein, especially red meat, can no longer be the main course for lunch or dinner if you are fighting disease and want to prevent a premature death. Diets high in saturated fat, calories and animal protein, like the Atkins diet, may help shed a few pounds in the short term but in the end a few pounds aren't worth the inflammation. In a recent study conducted over a year, blood vessel inflammation jumped 62 percent and vascular disease worsened in people on a high-protein diet.[30]

For people who have multiple risks for vascular disease, (a sedentary lifestyle, high cholesterol, hypertension, obesity, diabetes, metabolic syndrome or tobacco use), try to make meat and dairy products only 10 percent of your daily calories. For people facing vascular disease, try to abstain from animal protein, with the exception of egg whites and omega-rich fatty, cold-water fish. Frankly, I tell my patients that if you want to avoid another stent or bypass, or cure chronic angina and avoid a fatal heart attack, then you have to be uncompromising: *no meat*.

It's hard to believe that food changes can make a meaningful difference, but data from hundreds of studies show they can. The most prominent research project correlating animal protein with disease came from T. Colin Campbell, PhD's China Study. This study of diet and health led by Cornell and Oxford Universities, in concert with the China Nutritional Institute, surveyed a vast range of diseases, diet and lifestyle factors in rural and urban China.

The aim of the China Study was to investigate the role of nutrition, especially protein, in the development of disease. What they discovered was that safe proteins were from plants, including soy and wheat. Protein from animals promoted the development of certain cancers, including breast and colon cancer. Chinese who ate the most animal-based foods got the most chronic disease. People who ate the most plant-based foods were the healthiest and tended to avoid chronic disease. Evidence from the study strongly suggests that our diet should be 80 to 90 percent plant food.[31]

SECRET: To lose weight faster, eat raw foods such as apples, carrots, cauliflower, bell peppers and other whole fruits and vegetables. Snacking on crunchy foods slows the rate of digestion and provides thousands of disease-fighting nutrients.

Why We Don't Need So Much Meat

Animal protein and vegetable protein have similar effects on satiety. Don't worry about feeling hungry without meat in your diet. Protein stimulates glucagon, a hormone that tells the brain when it's time for the body to stop eating. If you're taking in adequate protein, regardless of the source, you'll trigger the action of glucagon. Glucagon has only one job, to mobilize stored carbohydrates in the liver that maintain stable blood sugar levels. As we discussed in the chapter on carbs, the brain depends on glucose for fuel. If you sustain stable blood sugar levels, you'll also maintain peak mental acuity, and you won't be hungry.

In America, we accept the inevitability of heart attacks, cancer and strokes, leading many of us to light up the grill and deny the ill-effects of our love affair with meat. A porterhouse steak is a great source of protein, but it also delivers fat, most of it saturated. Many popular American restaurants compete with each other by inflating portion sizes, offering three to four times the healthy portion size. Seafood is a leaner way to get your daily dose of protein than a big steak, and you'll get the heart-and-brain-healthy effects of omega-3 fatty acids. Salmon gives you protein without the saturated fat. Cooked lentils are loaded with protein, and practically no fat. Whole grains, nuts and beans are excellent sources of protein, and they have the added benefits of fiber, vitamins and minerals.

The China Study proved that a diet rich in animal protein has serious health consequences. "[The findings of the China Study] are not the results of a few isolated experiments. In most cases, they represent a summary of multiple studies, some of which are even many decades old," said Dr. Campbell. The findings are definitely enough evidence for us to *rethink* meat. We need about eight grams of protein for every twenty pounds of lean body weight to build and maintain our tissues. Eating a variety of healthy foods offers all the protein and amino acids your body needs.

SECRET: It takes 30-40 calories a day to maintain a pound of muscle; the more lean body mass you have, the faster your metabolism will be, and the greater number of calories you'll burn at rest.

CHAPTER 4
DIGESTING THE SOLUTION

Coronary artery disease, heart attack, stroke, obesity, insulin resistance and diabetes are closely related and 90 percent driven by diet. The U.S. leads the world in premature deaths from vascular disease, even though we have the best weapon to prevent, stop and reverse the caustic inflammation driving it. The Secret of the Non Diet is about using food selection—not dieting, calorie counting or portion control—to lose weight fast, keep it off, and end the course of a life-threatening disease. The secret is learning how to use the metabolizing of certain foods to your advantage. It is the only effective weapon we have to reverse the disease that is quietly killing our nation.

The diagnosis of a life-threatening illness can be a powerful motivator to make necessary changes in lifestyle. I don't know how many times I've heard a patient say that they were going to quit smoking or lose weight after a near-death experience involving an aneurysm, heart attack or stroke. Sometimes the decision comes after losing a loved one to the ravages of vascular disease. Other times the resolve grows when facing a lifetime of disability without changes. No one is invincible. Although the way many Americans continue to live, they seem to think so. Or perhaps we have been misled into thinking that medicine has all the solutions, especially when it comes to vascular disease. Stents, balloons, bypass and powerful statins don't prevent future strokes or heart attacks—the *"Easy Button"* doesn't work.

Nutrient-Friendly Foods

We derive nutrients from the vitamins, minerals, fibers and phytonutrients in natural foods. The term "phyto" originated from the Greek word for plant. Today 10,000 phytochemicals, disease-fighting plant chemicals, have been discovered. These nutrients have incredible effects on human physiology, including sweeping toxins out of cells, absorbing fat and cholesterol, preventing DNA damage which protects us from cancer, and offering protective benefits to colon and endothelial cells. Phytochemicals also improve our immune system and defenses against viruses and bacteria by detoxifying our cells. The goal for anyone trying to improve their health is to choose foods that have a high proportion of nutrients to calories.

Processed foods such as frozen french fries, canned fruits and white bread are stripped of fiber and valuable nutrients during the manufacturing process. They are basically empty calories with few nutrients. If you deep fry vegetables like okra and potatoes or overcook whole-wheat pasta, you'll lose important nutrients. Baking, boiling, steaming and stir-frying are better methods to protect the nutrients in foods. Grilling adds toxins that have been related to disease. If you're going to grill, wrap the food in foil.

As you begin to consume health-supporting, high-nutrient foods on a consistent basis, your appetite and cravings for lower-nutrient foods will decrease, and you'll eventually lose your addictions. You can feel the difference in as little as three weeks. It may not be easy to cut the umbilical cord to certain types of food, but then again, food isn't as addictive as nicotine or heroine. If you continue to eat a lot of foods that are high in calories and deficient in nutrients and fiber, and remain inactive, you might as well have a loaded gun pointed at your head. Americans too often put instant gratification and convenience ahead of nutrition.

The secret to preventing, stopping and reversing disease is to make starchy plant foods a *way of life*. We need to change the way we look at food. Food is fuel, and food is medicine. Diet is the most controllable cause of vascular disease and premature death, and only comprehensive changes will have a lasting impact on your health and well-being. Change starts with a personal decision, a resolution to improve the quality of your life. Consistency will strengthen your resolve, and time will cement it. It takes six weeks, on average, to break or make a habit.

Eat Like a Caveman?

We use a lot of brain cells selecting food. Evolutionary neuroscientists have even suggested that the way we evolved as hunters and gatherers promoted the development of our big brains—the biggest brains of any animal species. We rely on our prodigious senses of sight, smell, taste and touch, as well as memory and intelligence to guide and protect us. We shun sour and bitter tastes from infancy, and only learn how to like them through repeated conditioning, an innate aversion that was meant to protect us from poisoning. Human beings are the only animals that release a digestive enzyme that converts starch into simple sugars like glucose. Neural tissue depends on glucose.

The design of our anatomy—the olfactory nerves, teeth, tongue and taste buds, and the brain and gastrointestinal tract—is best suited for the slow digestion of raw starches and fibers, nutrient-dense products of nature that human beings have eaten for over a millennium. The typical low-carbohydrate, high-fat and low-fiber SAD diet is unsustainable in multiple ways, not just in terms of how we must eat to live.

Consider the cost to our U.S. treasury ($88 billion in agricultural subsidies over the last five years); to the environment (water, soil and air pollution, especially from our factory-style animal farms); and most of all, to the public health (an untold number). An estimated three out of four Americans die each year from serious diseases linked to diet. Cheap, plentiful food, it turns out, is unbelievably expensive in terms of lives. Diet-related disease costs the U.S. more health dollars than alcoholism, smoking and illegal drugs combined. What we choose to eat affects our health, the health of our children and the environment. The food industry depends on our ignorance and compliance for its continued success.

Non-Diet as a Way of Life

The considerable research of Dean Ornish, M.D., Paul Libby, M.D., Colin T. Campbell, Ph.D. and Caldwell Esselstyn, M.D. and many others have proven that a vegan diet of starchy complex carbohydrates is the best weapon for severe vascular disease, especially for patients with chronic angina or who are facing a second or third bypass surgery, stent or other procedure:

> The findings from the China Study indicate that the lower the percentage of animal-based foods that are consumed, the greater the health benefits—even when that percentage declines from 10% to 0% of calories. So it's not unreasonable to assume that the optimum percentage of animal-based products is zero, at least for anyone with a predisposition for a degenerative disease.[32]

Vegans eat only plants or products made from plants. Vegans following the Non-Diet way of eating also choose a greater percentage of starchy complex carbohydrates. If you have severe vascular disease or are recovering from a stroke, heart attack, angioplasty or other surgery, a loaded gun is pointing at your head. If you have trouble quitting meat, think about what the animal has to go through to end up on your plate. Visualize the slaughter of an animal.

A vegetarian diet is best suited for someone who doesn't have severe vascular disease, but has any number of the high risk markers described in Part II. These markers include high CRP or inflammation, LDL cholesterol and triglycerides, obesity, insulin resistance, diabetes, hypertension, tobacco use, poor aerobic fitness or chronic stress. In addition to starchy fruits and vegetables, legumes and whole grains, vegetarians can consume egg whites and low-fat dairy products. Anyone choosing plants instead of meat may want to take vitamin B12. We also recommend taking an omega-3 supplement and a multivitamin, but check with your doctor first for your specific nutrient needs.

Vegans and vegetarians can follow what some nutritionists call the 10 percent rule: the overwhelming majority, or 90 percent, of what you eat should follow the principles of the Non-Diet. The other 10 percent allows some wiggle room for omega-rich fish, birthday cake on birthdays, apple pie on the Fourth of July, and so on. But be forewarned, consuming even one high-fat meal such as a large slab of prime rib, creamy milkshake or pepperoni pizza can affect your heart, causing angina or EKG changes if you have vascular disease or diabetes. Studies have shown that a high-fat meal can bring on symptoms by raising triglycerides and reducing the heart's oxygen uptake.[33] As we learned in the chapter on fat, excess fat also damages the fragile endothelial cells lining our arteries. This causes prolonged endothelial dysfunction in the coronary arteries and microvascular vessels, a condition which reduces vital blood flow to the heart and brain.

What about Protein and Calcium?

If you're trying to prevent or reverse disease, you must avoid animal protein and seek plant-based protein instead. According to the Cleveland Clinic's Caldwell Esselstyn, M.D., "Compelling data from nutritional studies, population surveys, and interventional studies supports the effectiveness of a plant-based diet and aggressive lipid-lowering to arrest, prevent and selectively reverse heart disease."[34]

Both vegans and vegetarians can get all the protein, calcium and nutrients they need if they eat a variety of natural foods and prepare them in different ways—boiling, baking, steaming and "au natural." Frying adds fat. Americans consume about four servings of french fries a week. When prepared the right way, plant-based protein has no fat, lots of fiber, and virtually no cholesterol—the ideal disease-fighting combination.

We recommend a more flexible dietary option for people who have no risk factors for vascular disease, inflammatory disease or cancer, and want to stay healthy: "flexitarian." If you lean towards a vegetarian lifestyle but still eat beef, fish or poultry occasionally, you are a flexitarian. From our perspective, flexitarians should follow the secrets of the Non-Diet, selecting natural starchy foods first, then on occasion, adding meat. All animal products are low in the nutrients that protect against vascular disease and cancer: fiber, antioxidants, phytochemicals, folate, and plant proteins. Flexitarians should cut out soft drinks, processed snack foods and whole dairy products, including ice-cream, and save baked goods for special occasions to keep their arteries clean.

People think of diet as something that's short-term. But the word diet comes from the Greek root, "way of life." Hopefully by now, you'll see why the *type* of food you select is far more important than the amount of food you eat. As we discussed in the last three chapters, your body metabolizes the calories from carbohydrates, fats and proteins at different rates. It takes a lot more energy to burn off fat than it does to avoid fat calories in the first place.

Know Your Burn Rate

Your energy expenditure, or burn rate, is critical to your body weight. The number of calories your body uses, or burns, depends on your basic physiological needs, digestion and physical activity. Genetics plays a small role, mainly in determining your body shape. Your resting metabolic rate or RMR, the thermic effect of foods, temperature, and other stressors such as the frequency of meals, have the greatest influence on weight loss and maintenance. To determine the actual rate that your body burns calories just to maintain normal physiology, ask your doctor, nutritionist or physical therapist to assess your resting metabolic rate.

In general, you burn about 70 percent of calories at rest. Physical activity burns another 20 percent (unless you're a marathon runner), and the amount of calories burned during digestion depends on the food source. Resistant starch takes more energy and burns more calories during digestion. Winter squash, bran cereal, Navy beans and other complex carbohydrates increase the thermic effect of food which burns more calories as heat and energy. Even if we eat an excessive amount of carbohydrates, we burn more calories converting it into fuel, called glycogen, stored in our liver, kidneys and muscles.

If you have a fast metabolism, your body at rest will burn a greater number of calories. Men and tall persons tend to have a higher RMR. Lean body mass (organs, body water, bones and muscle) is metabolically active tissue. It takes 50 calories a day to maintain a pound of muscle. The more lean body mass you have, the greater your RMR will be.

If your RMR rate is slow, instead of burning calories, you will convert them to fat which takes only 3 calories a day to maintain. Turning up your RMR even slightly can have a major effect on your weight. You need to burn about 3,500 calories to lose one pound of fat. If you replaced just five pounds of body fat with five pounds of muscle, you would burn almost 55,000 more calories over a year, or 16 pounds of fat.

Everyone burns calories at a different rate. Genetics influence your RMR; studies on identical twins have found that twins tend to burn calories at the same rate. Geneticists have discovered a gene with special effects on RMR. Your RMR also slows down as you get older. For aging women, menopause will slow it down even more. Diet and exercise have the greatest effect on the rate of your metabolism.

Surprisingly, as you gain weight, your RMR increases because your body has to do more work to take care of the extra calories and pounds, but the increase in RMR is not enough to melt away the extra pounds. Eating small complex carbohydrate meals every 3-4 hours helps keep your metabolism high. Don't overeat, keep each meal between 300-400 calories with only 100-200-calorie snacks.

When you lose weight, your RMR also decreases because you'll need less energy to keep the body alive. For every three pounds of fat tissue you lose, you also lose a pound of muscle tissue. Using light weights and resistance exercises to build muscle mass will help you burn more calories, even after you've left the gym and have resumed your position on the couch.

Why Diets Fail

Commercial diet programs have to reduce portion sizes to cut down on the fat and calories in rich, high-fat entrees that appease the American palette. Dieting fails mainly because to keep the calories low, you have to reduce the amount of food you eat. After awhile, you'll walk-away feeling deprived, cheated and longing for the foods you gave up. Diets are short term solutions with long term consequences, including the loss of lean body mass. An evaluation of the most popular commercial diet plans, such as Atkins and Slim-Fast, revealed that the clients had a high probability of regaining 50 percent or more of lost weight in 1 to 2 years, despite the programs' considerable cost. The average weight lost was only three pounds.[35]

Contrary to popular belief, low-calorie diets make weight loss more difficult because deprivation slows your metabolism somewhat. When you quit dieting, your metabolism will remain low for at least a few weeks. If you return to the SAD during this period of adjustment, your weight could rebound. The "yo-yo" weight phenomenon is common among dieters.

Restricting carbohydrate calories may work in the short-term, allowing you to fit into that bikini, tuxedo or wedding dress, but in the long-term the diet will fail you. Even the worst diets for your heart may result in initial weight loss. Low-carbohydrate diets make no distinction between saturated and unsaturated fats and have been proven to elevate LDL cholesterol.[36]

The popular "detox" diets are nothing but clever marketing. Every day your powerful immune system, liver and kidneys rid your body of potential toxins without expensive flushing or cleansing products. These types of diets can be dangerous too, they promote a binge-purge mentality. To lose weight and successfully keep it off, you have to do it slowly and with the right type of food.

> **Fat-burning Fish Oil**
> Taking 1,000 mg of omega-3 fish oil each day for 2 months will increase your BMR, burning an estimated 200 calories daily.

The secret to successful weight-loss is to increase your RMR by using the different metabolic rates of food to your advantage. Eating a diet rich in complex carbohydrates can increase your RMR and help you lose weight slowly without feeling hungry. Your body only takes in 80 percent of the calories from complex carbohydrates; 20 percent are spent during digestion; another 35 percent are converted to glycogen stores in muscle and liver cells to be burned as heat or energy; and 15 percent of the calories are spent in the conversion to fat. In contrast, your body only uses up 3 percent of fat, and 10 percent of protein in metabolism.

The goal in weight loss is to get insulin to push sugars into your muscles as glycogen, instead of fat cells, where it can be an energy source. Glycogen is a polysaccharide that can be easily converted to glucose for energy. Building glycogen stores is one of the secrets to the Non Diet. Glycogen releases energy in the form of heat—the thermic effect of food. Insulin resistance can slow this process, this explains why a diabetic on a high protein diet cannot lose weight.

The body burns extra calories after a meal, in addition to the calories expended during rest. This calorie-burning is known as the thermic effect of food which represents 10-15 percent of the energy we burn on a daily basis. This is the best way to burn calories. The type of food you eat helps regulate this effect; some foods turn up our internal furnace and others don't at all.

Glycogen is made from natural sugars that come from carbohydrates. Broccoli, beans, whole-wheat spaghetti and multi-grain bread are good glycogen-builders. Butter, olive oil and beef cause a much slower calorie burn. The fiber or plant roughage from complex carbohydrates helps keep insulin levels in check too. The best foods for a calorie burn are foods high in fiber, and low in fat, such as apples, bananas, oranges, pears, asparagus, peas, broccoli, sweet potatoes; barley, kasha, pumpernickel bread and oatmeal.

Food can either supply you with nutrient-dense, fast-burning calories or fatty "empty" calories that you'll carry around your waist or hips. About half, or 40 percent, of the calories that Americans eat come from saturated fat in the form of processed foods and animal fats. About 250 different genes influence how your body metabolizes calories and regulates your appetite and satiety. Although heredity predisposes some to gain weight, what you eat and how often you exercise have the greatest influence on your size and shape. "Genetics loads the gun but environment pulls the trigger," as the old saying goes. To the degree that you adopt the Non-Diet way of life, you're going to lose weight, look and feel better, and best of all, you'll face a much lower risk of disease.

Food Selection, Not Deprivation

About 95 percent of Americans who attempt to diet and lose weight for their health end up gaining it back within a year. Why? They're dieting and not selecting. Supermarkets average 45,000 food selections, most of them packaged with elusive nutrition labeling and processed to stay on the shelf for months with the help of chemical additives. The average American has not been taught how to select and prepare whole foods that prevent and reverse disease.

Americans pay over $90 billion a year for the complications of obesity and that number is climbing. Yale professor Kelly Brownell, Ph.D. and Harvard Medical School professor, David Ludwig, M.D. have dedicated their careers to explore the cause and cure for eating and weight disorders. In a recent *Washington Post* editorial, they argued that the obesity epidemic has many causes, but the deterioration of our diet played a central role.[37] Yo-yo dieting, inactivity, poorly managed stress, and genetics contribute to obesity, but what you put in your mouth—or the mouths of your children—makes the biggest difference.

Over 4 billion people in the world don't have to face the devastating complications of vascular disease. What they have in common is a way of eating that includes lots of complex carbohydrate vegetables, legumes, whole grains and fruit. An oft-quoted study of autopsies done during the Korean and Viet Nam wars found that 70 percent of the American soldiers had evidence of coronary artery disease, but the Korean and Vietnamese soldiers of the same age had no evidence of vascular disease. After living with Americans and eating our SAD diet, the same Vietnamese soldiers developed vascular disease.

From Undernourishment to Overfed and Malnourished

One-hundred years ago, the poor of our country often lived with the misery of undernourishment and starvation. Today, low-income families are more likely to eat themselves to death than other economic classes. Obesity has replaced undernourishment. The likelihood of being overweight in the poorest 25 percent of the U.S. population is twice that of people in the highest quarter of economic class, according to Kelly Brownell, PhD., a professor of psychology, epidemiology and public health at Yale University.[38] If a parent is obese, statistics show their child will be too. The rate of overweight or obese minority children is 50 percent, compared to a rate of 35 percent among non-minority children.

We are leading our children down a path of disease earlier and earlier in their lives. Jay Olshansky, Ph.D., a professor of epidemiology and longevity researcher at the University of Illinois at Chicago, warned that the steady rise in life expectancy during the past two centuries may soon come to an end because of the unprecedented rate of obesity in children.[39] Several studies have found that the thinnest people live the longest. Research on centenarians, those who live into their 100s, confirmed that consuming a low-fat, low-calorie, plant-based diet extends lifespan. The China Study, the most comprehensive research project ever undertaken to explore the links between nutrition and disease, connected our SAD with vascular disease, certain cancers and other illnesses. Of the 10 leading causes of death in the United States, only three are *unrelated* to what we eat and drink.

Parents may not be aware that regular soft drinks, fruit drinks and fruit juices can also increase the odds of childhood obesity. Scientific studies have linked excessive juice and soft drink consumption to weight gain and obesity in children. Drinking just one sugary 12-oz. soda (150 calories) a day can add approximately 10 pounds of weight a year.[40]

Choosing to Live

And while everyone knows it is good to eat your vegetables, many people do not realize how easy it really is to consume five to nine servings of fruits and vegetables a day. For instance, just having a salad of leafy greens (two cups) with tomatoes and half a cup of broccoli totals four servings. If you had juice with breakfast, you're already up to five by lunchtime.

The Non-Diet offers an abundance of delicious, wholesome foods that can be part of many tantalizing gourmet recipes. Please see our section on "Recommended Reading" for references to recipe books that follow the Non-Diet philosophy.

I'm not for calorie counting—most of us don't have the time or bandwidth for it. Eating starchy, complex carbohydrates as much as you like, will help you lose weight and keep it off without feeling deprived. If you starve yourself, the appetite hormone leptin will drop too rapidly and you will feel tempted to overeat or binge. Your RMT will also slow. Dieters who eat several small meals a day will do better at sticking to a diet than dieters who skip meals. You need the energy from food to have the willpower to exert self-control in order to succeed on your diet. If you have no hunger or craving, and experience physical stamina and mental acuity, you know your last meal was nutritionally correct.

Taming Inflammation
Choose ginger, curry powder, grapes, garlic, celery, green tea and blueberries. Avoid trans fats, partially hydrogenated oils, simple sugars, meat and saturated fats.

If you eat a lot of refined-carbs like pasta, ice-cream and baked goods, it's much more difficult to control your total caloric intake. Blood levels of glucose and insulin also fluctuate more, leading to hunger. Insulin is one of the busiest hormones in your body. Many diet books have demonized insulin and carbohydrates because of the release of insulin into the bloodstream. Insulin is your friend when it is working properly. Severe carbohydrate restriction may cause you to lose weight quickly, but in the long run, you'll not only gain the weight back, you'll get a host of other health problems such as hypertension.

Good Carbs, Bad Carbs

Not that long ago, carbohydrates were the go-to for taste, comfort, convenience and energy. Today we have a different view. The *total* amount of carbohydrate in your diet isn't as important as the *type*. The data on increasing consumption of complex fiber-rich foods—whole grains, vegetables, legumes and fruits—to prevent or reverse vascular disease is compelling. A 2001 study reported in *Nutrition Reviews* found that eating just a handful of nuts five times weekly can reduce risk of vascular disease between 25 and 40 percent.

Consumption of simple carbohydrates leads to health problems. As we described earlier, different carbohydrate sources can have different effects on blood sugar, insulin and long-term health. Choosing good sources of slowly digesting carbohydrate foods will improve your health. Eating a lot of rapidly digested carbohydrates such as refined bread, tortillas or pasta will lead you down the path of insulin resistance, obesity, diabetes and premature death from vascular disease. Complex carbohydrates do not turn into body fat as easily, they are used up as energy.

As women age, menopause often causes weight-control problems; you'll have to carefully watch your diet and increase your physical activity to avoid gaining weight. Losing weight should be a gradual process. Anyone who's dieted, then overeaten to compensate, is familiar with the deprivation-binge-deprivation cycle, and with the weight gain that often accompanies it.

If you spend a little bit of time each day visualizing what you would like to look like or how you would like to change, it's more likely to happen. Research suggests that practicing visualization changes the physical structure of the neocortex, the "learning" part of the brain that helps you manage emotional stress. Visualization is similar to exercising, but the "muscle" is an area in the brain.

Some families collect their fat more on their abdomen than on their thighs or buttocks, but if eating a proper diet, it won't deposit there. Some of us have healthy bodies from birth, while others have bigger challenges. But what may seem like a genetic pattern of obesity may really be food or cooking habits passed down from generation to generation. Don't "settle" with the hand that was dealt to you, try to improve it.

What's For Dinner?

Many families gravitate toward foods that give them the most calories per dollar. According to a recent study by the American Dietetic Association, whole foods like fruits and vegetables not only cost more than fast food, but their prices are likely to rise as a result of inflation. What we serve at home has a great effect on the whole family. Fast food contains the worst fats, highly processed carbohydrates and little or no fiber. Choose low fat preparations such as baking, steaming, roasting, stewing or boiling instead of frying.

If you walk into most well-stocked supermarkets, which can have a bewildering number of choices, you'll see hundreds and hundreds of edible food-like substances that are masquerading as food. A lot of engineering goes into *processing* food to make it "healthy" after all the natural ingredients are stripped out.

If your child is obese, they may have an abnormal gene, and action must be taken quickly. Weight problems have been associated with certain chromosomes that trigger leptin, the appetite controller. When children have a healthy amount of body fat, leptin goes to the brain and slows down their appetite. Genes can lie as dormant as seeds on dry soil until certain kinds of foods come along. Studies on Asians and Native Americans revealed that, as they embraced the American diet, they became fatter and developed disease faster. Both ethnic groups evolved on a very different diet than they currently consume and, of course, their traditional levels of activity were much greater in the past than they are today. Immigrants from nations with low rates of vascular disease quickly acquired the illness after moving to America where the over-consumption of saturated fat, about 40 grams of fat versus the 12 to 15 grams of total fat per day eaten back home, is the cultural norm. Eating foods rich in saturated fat promotes artery-clogging cholesterol build-up.

If you cut saturated fats, you can lower the proportion of low-density lipoproteins (LDL) in your blood. Saturated fat hampers the effects of "good" cholesterol, high-density lipoprotein, or HDL, from doing its job: protecting the inner lining of your arteries from inflammatory agents that promote the build-up of plaque. Trans fats contain large numbers of free radicals, molecules with unpaired electrons that are highly reactive. Free radical damage in the arteries is thought to be an important factor in the initiation of plaque. But don't replace fat calories with carbohydrate calories in the form of refined flour and sugar. And don't forget to exercise.

Prosperous people who have leisure time are more likely to exercise than those who must work long hours to make ends meet. And we know that heart disease in westernized nations is more prevalent among the poor. You should exercise regularly, but watching the diet is more important. You have to burn 3,500 calories to lose one pound of weight, and that's not easy.

Food can maximize your potential for wellness and vibrancy, improving quality of life and preventing disease. Or, food can ruin your quality of life, promote chronic disease and leave you feeling run down and depressed. Poor life-style choices, genetics and aging contribute to a weakening of your health. You can alter this process by changing the type of food you eat, getting regular rest and exercising on a regular basis. A balanced lifestyle keeps inflammation at bay and your immune system strong. Comprehensive lifestyle changes can have a large impact on your energy level and your vascular health.

THE SECRETS OF THE NON-DIET

1. SECRET: All carbohydrates are not alike. Starchy, complex carbohydrates quell hunger and turn up our internal furnace, burning calories as heat and energy. High-sugar, high-fat, simple carbohydrates increase hunger, food addictions and cravings.

2. SECRET: The same starchy carbohydrates that prevent disease and premature death can stop and even reverse disease.

3. SECRET: The "resistant starch" in complex carbohydrates absorbs fat and cholesterol, and defies digestion while providing few calories and the feeling of fullness.

4. SECRET: Refined carbohydrates reduce the "good" HDL cholesterol and increase insulin levels, triglycerides, blood pressure and fat stores—proven culprits in the development of inflammation, obesity, diabetes and vascular disease.

5. SECRET: Foods that promote weight loss are high in complex carbohydrates which take more energy (calories) to break down. Your metabolism speeds up to process the critical nutrients of these foods. A faster metabolism can burn excess body fat.

6. SECRET: Consumption of complex carbohydrates helps the brain produce higher levels of serotonin which reduces your appetite and increases your feeling of well-being.

7. SECRET: Reducing saturated fat without reducing refined carbohydrates works against the goal to lose weight and prevent or reverse chronic disease.

8. SECRET: Saturated fats increase artery-clogging LDL-cholesterol. The unsaturated fats in oily fish, walnuts, flaxseeds and plant-based oils reduce LDL-cholesterol, inflammation and plaque within blood vessels.

9. SECRET: Trans fat offers what the Mayo Clinic calls "the cholesterol double-whammy:" it raises "bad" LDL-cholesterol and lowers "good" HDL-cholesterol. The greater the percentage of trans fat in a food product, the higher risk is for heart attack and stroke.

10. SECRET: Try to eliminate olive and other cooking oils while trying to lose weight, and then use them sparingly. Fish or a teaspoon of ground flaxseeds or walnuts offers the benefits of omega-3 fatty acids without all the fat of oil.

11. SECRET: Animal protein raises cholesterol while plant protein lowers it. Meat also raises artery-clogging saturated fat.

12. SECRET: To get the minimum amount of protein you need each day, balance your vegetables with beans and (if you're not on a diet) nuts.

13. SECRET: To lose weight faster, choose raw foods such as apples, carrots, cauliflower, bell peppers and other whole fruits and vegetables eaten raw. Snacking on crunchy foods slows the rate of digestion and provides thousands of disease-fighting nutrients.

14. SECRET: It takes 30-40 calories a day to maintain a pound of muscle. The more lean body mass you have, the faster your metabolism will be, and the greater number of calories you'll burn at rest.

THE VEGAN NON-DIET TO REVERSE DISEASE

Definition: A vegan is a person who does not eat meat or dairy.

Patient Profile: Severe vascular or microvascular disease; survivor of stroke, heart attack or heart failure; familial hyperlipidemia; cancer survivor; morbid obesity; anyone who wants to try to extend their lifespan.

Take action under your doctor's supervision:

✓ Start a new way of eating that focuses on *whole starches*: yams, potatoes, squashes, whole grains, legumes, yellow and green vegetables, and fruits.

  ✓ Steer clear of red meat, poultry, white flour, simple sugars, vegetable oils and all dairy products including milk, cream and cheese.

  ✓ Choose foods low in saturated fat and eliminate trans fatty foods such as baked goods. (See the list of fats on p. 22).

  ✓ Take a multivitamin, B12 and omega-3 fish oil supplements daily. (Calcium supplements are optional).

  ✓ Walk at least 30 minutes, 6 days a week; exercise feeds a diseased heart, lowers blood pressure and blood sugar, and fights depression.

  ✓ Practice mind-body techniques daily such as prayer, visualization, yoga, positive thinking, or meditation to reduce stress, increase energy and maintain mental acuity.

  ✓ No smoking. Limit alcohol intake to one glass of red wine weekly.

Rudy Kachmann, M.D.

THE VEGETARIAN NON-DIET TO DROP WEIGHT AND/OR REVERSE DISEASE

Definition: A vegetarian is a person who does not eat meat.

Patient Profile: Overweight; metabolic syndrome or diabetes; smoker; hypertension; non-familial hyperlipidemia; sedentary lifestyle; high stress; anyone who wants to try to extend lifespan or improve physical appearance, energy and stamina.

Take action under your doctor's supervision:

✓ Start a new way of eating that focuses on *whole starches*: yams, potatoes, squashes, whole grains, legumes, yellow and green vegetables, and fruits.

  ✓ Choose primarily plant-based foods. Avoid red meat, poultry, white flour, simple sugars, vegetable oils and whole dairy products including milk, cream and cheese.

  ✓ Choose foods low in saturated fat and eliminate trans fatty foods such as baked goods. (See the list of fats on p. 22).

  ✓ Take a multivitamin, B12 and omega-3 fish oil supplements daily. (Calcium supplements are optional).

  ✓ Exercise at least 30 minutes, 4 days a week; exercise lowers blood pressure and blood sugar, and fights depression.

  ✓ Practice mind-body techniques daily such as prayer, visualization, yoga, positive thinking, or meditation to reduce stress, increase energy and maintain mental acuity.

  ✓ No smoking. Limit alcohol intake to one glass of red wine daily.

Rudy Kachmann, M.D.

THE FLEXITARIAN RX TO MAINTAIN OPTIMAL HEALTH

Definition: A flexitarian is a semi-vegetarian; someone who eats primarily plant-based foods and limits consumption of red meat and whole dairy.

Patient Profile: A semi-vegetarian lifestyle works well for people with no risk factors who want to maintain normal weight, remain healthy or improve physical appearance, energy and stamina.
Take action under your doctor's supervision:

✓ Start a new way of eating that focuses more on whole starches: yams, potatoes, squashes, whole grains, legumes, yellow and green vegetables, and fruits.

✓ Choose primarily plant-based foods. Limit red meat, poultry, white flour, simple sugars, vegetable oils and whole dairy products including milk, cream and cheese.

✓ Choose foods low in saturated fat and eliminate trans fatty foods such as baked goods. (See the list of fats on p. 22).

✓ Take a multivitamin and omega-3 fish oil supplements daily.

✓ Exercise at least 30 minutes, 4 days a week; exercise lowers blood pressure and blood sugar, and fights depression.

✓ Practice mind-body techniques daily such as prayer, visualization, yoga, positive thinking, or meditation to reduce stress, increase energy and maintain mental acuity.

✓ No smoking. Limit alcohol intake to one glass of red wine daily.

Rudy Kachmann, M.D.

PART II:
OLD MYTHS, NEW RESEARCH ON VASCULAR DISEASE

CHAPTER 5

INFLAMMATION: THE HEART OF THE MATTER

From a purely mechanical standpoint, the heart is a pump. And what a pump it is. The four-chambered muscle, weighing only 10 ounces, pumps over 100 gallons of blood an hour through the body's circulatory system of arteries, veins, arterioles and capillaries. Every tissue in the body depends on the heart for survival. During a typical heartbeat, the heart contracts to push blood out to the rest of the body and then relaxes to fill up with returning blood. Pressure inside the heart muscle, not electrical signals from the brain, forces the cardiac valves to open and shut like a water valve—*lub-dup, lub-dup*. The heart beats 35 million times a year, nearly 2.5 billion times during an average lifespan.

You may think that the brain controls the heart, but in Chapter 11, we discuss how the heart often functions independently from the brain. The sinoatrial (SA) node is the heart's internal generator that controls the heart's rhythm, and is one of the reasons why life ceases without a heart, but can continue for a period of time without a functioning brain. The heart perceives changes in blood pressure, viscosity, warmth and biochemical composition with tiny sensory receptors, sensing devices that sit on top of its cells, and by means of hormones and other "informational substances," in addition to electrical signals from the nervous system and brain.

Blood circulates throughout our fluid 60,000-mile circulatory system at least once a minute, sometimes at the rate of 10 miles per hour, depending on our body weight and activities. Billions of red blood cells deliver oxygen to all the trillions of cells in our body. The heart pumps the oxygen-rich blood to the brain and extremities through the arteries, and transports the oxygen-poor blood from the veins to the lungs to gain oxygen. Arteries have thick muscular walls to help withstand and control the blood pressure.

The coronary arteries that run on the surface of the heart have three major branches. The right coronary artery supplies blood mainly to the right side of the heart and the lungs. The left coronary artery, which branches into the left anterior descending and the circumflex arteries, supplies blood to the left side of the heart, the main pumping chamber that pumps blood to the rest of the body.

Until quite recently, the most critical forms of vascular disease were considered to involve these major arteries. However, advanced diagnostics and new research on "female-pattern" vascular disease—the topic of Chapter 3—has highlighted the crucial involvement of the microcirculation (small and microscopic vessels) in many vascular conditions.

Bonfire of the Arteries

An explosion of new research is changing our view of the relationship between inflammation and vascular disease. Inflammation is a functional immune reaction to fever, injury and infection, but it can also be a dysfunctional and damaging process, especially to our arteries and vital organs. The most common inflammatory triggers include LDL cholesterol, obesity, metabolic syndrome, diabetes, hypertension, smoking, a high-saturated fat diet and the toxic biochemicals of chronic stress, depression and anger.[41] Scientists and doctors have discovered that inflammation is the driving force in all stages of vascular disease, from the fatty-streaks to the life-threatening blood clots of heart attack and stroke.

Peter Libby, M.D., a professor at the Harvard Medical School and Chief of Cardiovascular Medicine at Brigham and Women's Hospital, is one of the pioneers in revealing how inflammation causes atherosclerosis, heart attack and stroke. Dr. Libby argues that we can no longer compare coronary arteries and their branches to "inanimate conduits" analogous to pipes. Endothelial cells are teeming with bioactive substances that regulate cellular growth, vascular tone, blood coagulation and inflammatory responses. Arteries are dynamic tissues, exchanging chemical signals with the brain, heart and immune system, and living in rhythmic movement to mediate the needs of our body.[42]

About five percent of the blood from each heart beat enters the coronary arteries, raising the odds of tiny arterial tears. Excess LDL cholesterol floating in the bloodstream can collect on these tears. Fatty-streaks of inflammatory substances attack the accumulating lipids. Over time these "lesions" can grow into pimple-like plaques that reduce the arteries' elasticity and interfere with blood flow, but only 5-10 percent of heart attacks and strokes are due to narrowed arteries. The overwhelming majority of vascular events are due to the rupture of plaque that triggers an immune system response to "heal" the lesion, including blood clotting which can block blood flow.[43] Like one of the definitions of *inflammation*, the arteries are "on fire."

The thin, flat endothelial cells lining the arteries play a vital role in dividing blood from tissue and tissue from blood. Small particles of LDL cholesterol can slip through the thin layer of cells and into the deeper layers of tissue, triggering the development of plaque and an inflammatory response that can fester for years. People with vascular disease might have one or two plaques, or dozens distributed throughout their arteries. Women are more likely to develop plaque that spreads like peanut butter within the arterial tissue, narrowing the circumference of the artery.

Several large research projects, including the Women's Health Study, a long-term national health study that explores strategies to prevent chronic disease, found that 50 percent of the participants who developed vascular disease had high levels of the inflammatory marker CRP, even though their LDL cholesterol levels were normal.[44] Inflammation was the culprit. As many as 35 million Americans have normal lipid profiles but high levels of inflammation damaging their arteries. Paul Ridker, M.D., another pioneer, was one of the primary researchers in the women's study who urged doctors to focus on an aggressive reduction of inflammation through lifestyle changes with diet and exercise at the top of the list. Too many strokes and heart attacks strike without warning, and too many medical therapies meant to avert such events fail. Most heart attacks aren't caused by the fatty build-up of plaque that closes-off an artery.

After completing the New York City Marathon, Matthew P. Hardy, a 50-year-old research scientist and competitive runner, returned to his Manhattan apartment, collapsed, and died. A spokeswoman for the New York City Medical Examiner's Office blamed "an acute thrombotic occlusion of the left anterior descending coronary artery." A clot in his coronary artery had sent him into cardiac arrest:

> Hardy was no novice to marathon running. He completed the New York marathon every year between 1995 and 2005, clocking between 3 hours 47 minutes 21 seconds and 5:29:10. On Sunday, he finished in 4:48:21 before going home and complaining of labored breathing.[45]

IN FOCUS: THE PATHOLOGY OF VASCULAR DISEASE

On a clinical level, several varieties of highly-adaptable cells, enzymes and molecules play a role in the complex pathology of vascular disease but scientists have studied LDL cholesterol's role more than any other inflammatory trigger. Similar to the process that spoils milk, lipids accumulating inside the wall of the artery undergo oxidation and their proteins undergo both oxidation and glycation (binding by sugars), one of the key chemical reactions that sets off a chain of events leading to the build-up of plaques.

When immune cells living in the arterial tissue discover the modified LDL, they migrate to the spleen or lymphoid tissues where they activate the growth of white blood cells—helper T-cells, killer T-cells and B-cells. Endothelial and smooth muscle cells in the artery also secrete chemokines to attract monocytes that defend endothelial cells by releasing cell-destroying toxins. Neutrophils also move in to obliterate anything in their path. T lymphocytes are the immune system's "special agents" that track-down and destroy any stragglers. Oxidation transforms the monocytes into macrophages that gobble-up LDL as if it were a virus or bacteria. Macrophages play multiple roles in inducing the development and rupture of plaque.

If macrophages eat too much oxidized LDL, they lose their ability to identify foreign invaders and self-destruct into foam cells, dumping their toxic waste into the blood vessel wall, amplifying the inflammatory activity. Smooth muscle cells finally arrive to coat the accumulating lipid core with a protective cap. The end result is a plaque filled with multiplying white blood cells, LDL cholesterol, toxic foam and dead or dying macrophages.

Substance Matters, Not Size

Plaques vary in size, quantity and composition. Older, calcified plaques large enough to be picked up on angiography tend to be more stable, only causing an estimated two to three out of 10 heart attacks. Over the past decade, cardiologists discovered that the substance inside the plaque matters more than the size. Smaller plaques with soft, lipid-dense cores have thin, fibrous caps which are vulnerable to rupture—and harder to detect with standard diagnostics. To visualize soft plaque directly, a procedure called CT angiography with the injection of dye is done.

Anything that increases stress, blood pressure, heart rate or the force of the heart beat can tear or rupture a vulnerable plaque. Not all vulnerable plaques rupture. If the cap ruptures, a cascade of events follows. Inflammatory substances (growth factors, collagen, white blood cells and lipids) spill out into the blood stream, triggering white blood cells that summon platelets to seal the rupture or "infection." A clot forms with the sticky debris, blocking blood flow from the artery. If the clot blocks a coronary artery, a heart attack occurs. A clot blocking a cerebral artery leading to the brain causes a stroke.

Most of the heart consists of oxygen-hungry muscle fibers that quickly begin to die (infarct) without oxygen-rich nutrients. Inflammatory cells rush to the site of the infarction and signal the production of a massive amount of oxygen free radicals that further destroy heart tissue and often cause a chaotic rhythm that cannot circulate blood. Sudden cardiac death ensues without medical intervention.

One-third of the people who have a heart attack, or 500,000 people, each year never make it to the hospital and die from sudden cardiac death, according to Steven E. Nissen, M.D., Chairman of the Department of Vascular Medicine at the Cleveland Clinic. But a sudden, catastrophic heart attack isn't the fate of most people who have lingering vascular disease. They may have several silent attacks or minor ones that require stenting. Or they may develop congestive heart failure and experience a diminished quality of life.

Common Inflammatory Diseases

- Alzheimer's
- Asthma
- Cancer (mouth, esophageal, lung, breast, liver, stomach, pancreatic, colon, rectum, ovarian, endometrial, prostate)
- Chronic Obstructive Pulmonary Disease (COPD)
- Coronary Artery Disease
- Crohn's Disease
- Grave's Disease
- Lupus
- Microvascular Disease
- Multiple Sclerosis
- Obesity (see Chapter 6)
- Ulcerative Colitis
- Pelvic Inflammatory Disease
- Psoriasis
- Rheumatoid Arthritis
- Type 2 diabetes

Systemic or body-wide inflammation is hard to detect. Swelling, redness and tenderness to the touch are obvious signs of inflammation in muscles and joints. Two good ways to measure the inflammation inside arteries include checking your homocysteine and C-reactive protein levels. Ask your doctor for the test.

Collateral Damage

A major benefit of the inflammatory response, the body's defense against infection and foreign infiltration, is righting the countless wrongs that threaten our lives. But sometimes the very same complex immune functions that ensure our survival also lead to our downfall. Prolonged or chronic inflammation leads to the simultaneous destruction and healing of arterial tissue, a lingering collateral damage from the body's disease-fighting response. Only a few years ago, scientists and doctors thought of the disease as a lipid storage disease: excess LDL cholesterol would accumulate on the surface of arteries, obstructing blood-flow and eventually causing a heart attack or stroke. With advanced imaging diagnostics such as MRA and ultrasound technology, cardiologists can detect arterial disease at earlier stages, well before changes to the lumen (outside) of the artery become detectable. We now understand that plaque develops deep within, rather than on, arterial walls. And we've learned that vascular events rarely result from older, calcified plaques viewable via angiography.

Vascular disease is primarily an inflammatory process of irritation, injury, healing and re-injury inside the blood vessels. The sum total of these recent findings has led to a new diagnosis and treatment paradigm in which you are the key player. The first step is to know your numbers. Asking your doctor to check the vascular markers for inflammation in your blood such as CRP can lead to early treatment and reversal, or prevention of life-threatening complications.

The second step is to stabilize vulnerable plaque by reducing arterial inflammation through diet, exercise, losing weight and if needed, statin therapy, rather than controlling the size of the plaque through short-term procedures that don't prevent a future heart attack or stroke. Patients feel they can eat whatever they want as long as they take a statin drug to lower cholesterol, but "powerful" statin drugs only reduce plaque by about five to seven percent. Following the Non-Diet program can have as much of an effect on cholesterol levels as modern medicine does. You are your own best friend or worst enemy in the fight against vascular disease.

CHAPTER 6
NEW INSIGHTS INTO BRAIN ATTACKS

The 18-hour work day was coming to a close, or so I thought. I had just finished admitting a 10-year-old boy in critical condition to the intensive care unit. A pick-up truck driven by the boy's father had been rear-ended by a man who was under the influence of alcohol and speeding. The impact of the crash severed the young boy's spinal cord. He could no longer walk, move or breathe on his own. His injuries were so severe in fact that nothing less than a sheer will to live was keeping him alive. His father, a local triathlete who had survived the accident without a scratch, was out of his mind with anger and grief.

It had been a record day of misery after three miserable nights of work-interrupted sleep, but as I sat finishing my paperwork in the pods of the ER, Cooper, a white-bearded radiologist who liked to wear flashy bow ties, held up a CTA (Computer Tomography Angiogram) film in front of my eyes and pointed to a large blood clot clogging the anterior cerebral artery of a brain.

The brain belonged to Teddy, a large African-American who was lying in the ICU. Teddy was 36 years old, married and the father of three young children. He was also the owner of a successful auto shop on the north side of town. Earlier that day, his wife Nadine found him lying unconscious on the bathroom floor and immediately called 911.

I walked into the nurses' station and asked my nurse and assistant, Robert, for Teddy's chart. Robert orchestrated my clinic visits and surgery schedule, but more importantly, he was walking Prozac in a field of medicine that could be depressing. He had long dreadlocks, a soothing baritone voice, and a big, broad smile. His striking 6'2" stature and unassuming manner made people forget about the gravity of their circumstances, if only for a moment. He never talked in front of a patient as if he or she wasn't there, even if the patient was unconscious, comatose or under anesthesia. Like me, Robert believed that a patient's unconscious awareness had the power to influence the outcome of surgery and life-and-death situations.

When I opened the sliding glass door of the ICU, I could see the mountainous profile of a man lying beneath the sterile-white hospital sheets. His wife looked up at me from her chair before roaming her eyes over the room's web of wires, beeping monitors and flashing lights with an unmistakable look of bewilderment. Nurses and aides surrounded Teddy, taking blood, attaching monitors, inserting an intravenous line and a catheter. Teddy could move his left side but could not speak. His right side was paralyzed, his mouth drooping. I introduced myself as Dr. Rudy Kachmann, the on-call neurosurgeon, while Robert checked his IV, blood oxygenation, heart rate and blood pressure to look for any signs of distress.

I began my neurological exam. Teddy's eyes moved symmetrically and his pupils reacted when I flashed a pinpoint of light in his eyes with my penlight. He could answer a few brief questions with eye contact, but he had no recall of objects that I had asked him to remember just a few minutes earlier. He flinched when I stuck a needle in the big toe of his left foot; however, he had no reflexes or sensations in his right foot.

Teddy's lab work revealed high levels of CRP and blood fats called triglycerides, and low levels of high-density lipoprotein, the good cholesterol. He also had enough insulin and glucose in his blood to interfere with how his kidneys work. His blood pressure was out of control. All the clinical evidence was there: Teddy was having a stroke— a sudden blockage of blood flow to the brain. Strokes, not automobile accidents, are the number one cause of adult disability in the U.S. Deaths from strokes have abated with preventive care and better rehabilitation.

Brain Matters

The essential biochemical processes that keep the complex circuitry of the brain humming—the breakdown of glucose into its component parts—demand a great deal of fresh oxygen pumped from the heart and lungs. During any mental or physical activity, such as writing a sentence or solving a math problem, blood flow and glucose metabolism accelerate in the appropriate brain region. The brain does not keep these vital substances on reserve. Without oxygen-rich blood coursing through the cerebral arteries at every instant, brain cells begin to suffocate within five to 10 minutes, and the mechanisms that control involuntary functions such as breathing, or voluntary functions such as thinking and moving, may begin to falter. Ischemia, cell suffocation from the lack of blood flow, snuffs out a life an overwhelming majority of the time.

The brain is a complex biological organ of great computational capability that constructs our sensory experiences, regulates our thoughts and emotions and controls our actions. The brain processes information through conscious thought and unconsciously through nerve systems that control essential functions like heart rate, temperature control, digestion and balance. With imaging scans, neurologists can even follow the traces of thought as it travels through various divisions of the brain. To coordinate the seamless integration of thought and movement, far-flung parts of the body must be in constant communication with one another.

Over one trillion cells comprise the body's nervous system, which reaches into the body to serve the needs of our individual human experience. Our nervous system interacts with every other system in our body. In the same way that all of our cells need oxygen transported by the circulatory system, all of our tissues and organs need to transmit information to and from the brain and nervous system. Nerve impulses from the body to the brain affect our reasoning, emotions and choices.

Our brain and body use the nerves in the central nervous system (CNS) and autonomic nervous system (ANS), hormones and other "informational substances" to communicate. Most of this activity takes place at a subconscious level. Sometimes what we experience comes from activity in specialized brain regions; other times chemicals in our body change our experience. "The range of information conveyed to the brain is wider than expected, from the concentration of chemical molecules to the contractions of muscles anywhere in the body," said neurologist Eric Kandel, M.D.[46]

Our three-pound gray wonder sitting on top of our head can store over 25 million books on its memory shelves; a bookshelf that would be 500 miles long and a library even bigger than the Library of Congress. The computational rate of the brain, how fast it can process information, surpasses the speed of the world's largest supercomputer by tens of thousands of trillions per second. The amount of information it processes at once—visual images, sounds, touch, emotions and memories, not to mention all the "stuff" that happens without our conscious knowledge—is unknown.

On a cellular level, we are busy, busy creatures. The adult brain contains over 10 billion neurons and another 100 billion support cells that form over 100 trillion connections with each other. Every few weeks, neurons, the primary cells of the nervous system, die and replace themselves. Neurons don't multiply, however. The majority of the neurons in your brain and nervous system are as old as you are. What changes with time and experience are the small gaps between the neurons—the synaptic connections. A cubic millimeter of cortical tissue, the size of the "0" on your cell phone, holds about a billion synapses. Any single neuron in the brain can have 100 to 10,000 synaptic connections.

Genes may determine our potential, but synaptic connections determine who we are. Synapses are the primary information channels in the brain. Their particular pattern and the information stored within them are the keys to your personal identity. Neurologist Joseph LeDoux, M.D. goes as far as to say that we are who we are because of our synaptic connections in his book, *Synaptic Selves*. Experience continually remodels our neural connections. With the aid of powerful molecular microscopes and advanced photographic techniques, neuroscientists can see synapses change after repetition of a certain activity or routine.

Practice, whether it's playing golf or tennis, composing music, using a foreign language or performing yoga and brain surgery, hopefully not at the same time, literally changes the structures of the brain. Practice does not make perfect. The brain is incapable of planning the same movement each and every time. But whenever you participate in an activity that requires persistent visual or physical repetition, neural pathways grow and reorganize, forming a template for that activity. Without purpose, weaker synaptic connections wither away: *use it or lose it*. Remaining socially connected and keeping the brain stimulated by reading, doing puzzles and learning new things will protect the brain against dementia. Throughout a person's lifetime, synapses continually alter their strength, adding an extra layer of complexity to the brain's operations and differentiating the human brain from "hardwired" machines like the Apple computer.

The corpus callosum, the dividing line that separates the right and left hemispheres of the brain, weaves together the two sides of the brain. Each hemisphere processes information in different ways. Our right hemisphere controls the left half of the body, and our left hemisphere controls the right half. The right frontal cortex creates our perceptual skills, including the perception of The Big Picture, the awareness that we are connected to something greater than ourselves. Creativity, free-thinking and spontaneity are predominantly right-brain activities.

Empathy, intuition and understanding the subtle cues of "body language" are also right-brain processes.

Abstract and verbal powers are more dominant on the left side of the brain. The left hemisphere of the brain processes information in a linear and methodical way. Moments are divided into the past, present and future. When I slide into the driver's seat of my car, it is the left side of my brain that processes that I must put the key in the ignition before the car will run. Forming sequences, critical judgments, analysis and deductive reasoning are left-brain tasks. Language and music also predominantly occur in the left hemisphere.

Any damage to the brain's hemispheres can radically change how you perceive the world around you. A stroke in the right hemisphere can affect your ability to read emotional cues, leaving the left hemisphere to interpret everything literally, like a young child often does. If I remark that I don't know what he has "up his sleeve" to someone with a damaged right hemisphere, they may interpret what I said as having something hidden up their sleeve. The functions of our brain hemispheres complement one another.

When a Stroke Attacks

A sudden interruption of brain activity, such as a sudden loss of blood oxygen, can impact normal functions that we take for granted. Neurons are adaptable and can undergo changes in utility and shape that allow them to take on the functions of nearby damaged cells in a process called neural plasticity, but a stroke causes irreversible changes. Damaged brain cells cannot regenerate to any significant extent, only about two percent. Recovery of mental and physical functions requires the arduous work of rehabilitation and belief in the plasticity of the brain—its ability to repair its neural circuitry.

A steely determination, positive attitude and sense of humor go a long way toward recovery. "Never underestimate the human spirit and the will to get better," said stroke survivor and author, Julia Fox Garrison:

> In my ongoing recovery, I picture myself as any professional—an athlete, an actor, a musician—who strives to achieve by practice, hard work, and determination. Like a tennis player working on her backhand, I am constantly working on my gait or on trying to control my spastic left arm.[47]

Warning Signs of Stroke
S = Sudden difficulty speaking
T = Tingling in arm, hand or leg
R = Recall, memory problems
O = Off-balance or dizzy
K = Killer headache
E = Eyes blurry or dim vision

A stroke occurs when blood flow to part of the brain is suddenly interrupted, which is why we call it a "brain attack." The brain depends on two major sets of vessels to bring fresh blood, carrying oxygen and nutrients, from the heart and lungs: the carotids located in the front of the neck, and the vertebral arteries in the back of the neck. The jugular veins and others take away blood carrying carbon dioxide and cellular waste. Arteries that carry blood into the brain taper into smaller and smaller vessels to feed specific areas of the brain. These smaller vessels can become blocked by a blood clot—the cause of stroke 85 percent of the time. Slightly less than 20 percent of strokes are hemorrhagic, a problem that occurs when a blood vessel bursts and causes bleeding in the brain. Hemorrhagic strokes are more likely to occur in people with chronic high blood pressure.

From a clinical perspective, stroke is a neurological deficit resulting from cessation of blood flow through one of the vessels supplying the brain with vital nutrients and oxygen. The deficit must last more than 24 hours for the episode to be diagnosed as a stroke. A few years ago, doctors prescribed bed rest at home for a mild stroke such as a transient ischemic attack (TIA). Although TIAs usually clear up within a few minutes or an hour, today doctors consider TIAs a "brain attack" that requires immediate, emergency intervention by trained medical professionals.

Anyone suffering symptoms of stroke should call 911. In research from Oxford University, doctors found that patients treated within 24 hours of a TIA cut their risk of having a more serious stroke in the next three months by 80 percent.[48] Neurologists or neurosurgeons can place a catheter in the artery of the groin, feed it up to the artery blocked in the brain and administer clot-busting medications, saving the brain from more severe, irreversible injuries. This treatment is available in most medium-size hospitals, but even if you live in a small town, you should go to the local ER, where typically you can be airlifted to a larger hospital. Treatment needs to be administered within the first few hours of the initial presentation of symptoms.

Small strokes are a warning signal for an impending stroke like angina or chest pain may be for an impending heart attack. When brain cells die as a result of stroke, the resulting injury to the brain is called a cerebral infarction. Denial or delay in treatment can cost cognitive and motor skills, or even a life.

Recognizing Stroke

A bystander can recognize a stroke by asking three simple questions. Ask the person to:
1) SMILE.
2) SPEAK.
3) RAISE THEIR ARMS.
If he or she has trouble with ANY of these tasks, call 911.

About two-thirds of people who have a stroke have some resulting disability and require rehabilitation. Treatments for stroke are inexact. Long-term recovery largely depends on the body's own ability to heal itself. But without the clot-busting medication that Teddy quickly received in the ER, and the care he continued to receive in the ICU, more severe brain damage, and even death, was still a possibility.

One of the brain's most vital jobs is to send signals from the brain stem to the respiratory system to keep the muscle of the diaphragm moving. Interruption of these signals and collapse of vital function is one of the most common manifestations of stroke that kills approximately 20 percent of its victims. Worldwide, nearly 15 million people have a stroke each year. Stroke is one of the leading killers in the developed world, trailing only vascular disease and cancer in the United States.[49]

Anatomy of Brain Attack

Strokes typically occur when a buildup of plaque ruptures from the inner wall of an artery, triggering the formation of a blood clot that is propelled up into the brain through the neck and head's artery system. Signs and symptoms of stroke vary, depending upon which artery is blocked and what parts of the brain can no longer function. Sensory loss, facial numbness, visual and language disturbances, paralysis on one side of the body, a sudden severe headache and difficulties in balance are some of the more common manifestations of stroke. One of my patients compared her symptoms to having a shot of Novocain that numbed the entire left half of her body.

Strokes mainly involve narrowing or blockage of the middle cerebral artery (MCA), which supplies blood to the lateral surface of the cerebral hemisphere, and the brain centers that lie deep beneath the cortex. In Teddy's case, a large blood clot had lodged into his left anterior cerebral artery (ACA). The ACA extends upward and forward into the brain from the neck's carotid artery. Strokes in the ACA can distort the thinking part of the brain, disturb memory and personality, and even paralyze the side of the body opposite to the obstruction. For the most part, the right side of the brain controls the left side of the body, and the left side of the brain controls the right side of the body.

The brain is an exquisitely sensitive and hungry organ. Brain metabolism ceases when blood supply is cut off for more than 30 seconds. After one minute, nerve function may cease. After five minutes, lack of oxygen to the brain initiates a chain of events that may result in stroke: local arterial dilation; a decrease in blood flow; brain swelling; and death to the affected brain tissue. If the interruption of blood flow is sufficiently prolonged and a portion of the brain dies, the tissue first softens, then liquefies, and a cavity or hole in the brain forms. Over time, scar tissue fills in part of the hole and new blood vessels form.

The immediate reaction of brain tissue to ischemia, or lack of blood flow, is swelling. When the energy cycle of the brain breaks down, fluid begins to accumulate within the membrane of brain cells and eventually leaks into the surrounding brain tissue. Loss of consciousness and coma are possibilities when brain swelling causes severe intracranial pressure that creates even more pressure on the brain. When stroke occurs in younger people, it can be more damaging because as the body ages, the brain shrinks a little. Older people have room to accommodate some swelling inside their skulls.

If severe neurological deterioration occurs, such as a blown eye pupil, there may be a need for emergency craniotomy to relieve pressure on the brain. A "blown pupil" refers to the eye's sudden dilation and loss of ability to constrict in response to light. It can be a devastating, clinical sign in stroke, and may foreshadow an impending brain herniation or another catastrophe. Typically, a patient with a blown pupil is whisked off to the operating room (OR) for an emergency craniotomy during this procedure a neurosurgeon removes a very large portion of the patient's skull on the affected side of the brain and opens the dura, the lining that surrounds the brain, to relieve pressure on the brain. This helps in some cases, but not all.

When cellular injury and swelling occur during trauma or a stroke, neurons, or brain cells, release powerful amino acids that break down brain tissue in an effort to relieve pressure. Brain bleeding that causes swelling of surrounding tissues requires immediate neurosurgical intervention with the insertion of an intracranial pressure monitor and the administration of hyperosmotic agents, such as mannitol, to remove fluid from the brain tissues.

Although most strokes are bland—bloodless—bleeding into the brain can occur which may be minor or major. Neurologists take care of the bland strokes. Neurosurgeons often have to intervene in the major strokes that bleed into the brain. Bleeding can occur through dying brain tissue or when the original blood clot in the artery breaks up and migrates, restoring blood flow to the injured brain too soon. Like a garden hose that has been cut off from the water supply for a short period of time, blood pressure in the blocked artery is much higher than normal. When a blood clot in the artery breaks up and migrates, restoring blood flow to the injured brain tissue, bleeding into the surrounding membranes can occur like water spraying out from a garden hose.

The initial stroke kills neurons fed by the blocked artery. A second brain death occurs when neurons release noxious chemical agents (excitory amino acids) that kill surrounding brain tissues, resulting in a larger stroke volume and intracranial pressure. In the worst case scenario, the increased pressures affect the good brain and result in herniation of the brain through the skull, injuring the brain stem and vital tissues, quickly resulting in death. Neurologists and neurosurgeons treat a large stroke with mannitol and other osmonic agents to immediately reduce the brain swelling. In extreme cases, where the swelling isn't controllable, we perform a craniotomy.

Only one quarter of stroke patients die, half regain function, and another quarter of patients need long-term care. Neurologists, neurosurgeons, vascular surgeons, cardiologists and radiologists are some of the specialists who overlap in the prevention and treatment of the underlying pathology of the majority of strokes—atherosclerosis (vascular disease). Ultrasound, angiogram and other sensitive diagnostics are used to demonstrate and diagnose the disease.

Striking at an Early Age

A popular misconception is that stroke is a disease of the elderly. It is true that most stroke victims are older and, as the country's population ages, the incidence of stroke is going up. But stroke in people younger than 50 is also increasingly common. Men and women are about equally likely to have a stroke, but women have a greater risk of dying from one. African-Americans are almost twice as likely to suffer a stroke as are whites. We're seeing people with stroke in their 30s and 40s because of vascular disease, hypertension, diabetes and the prevalence of our sedentary lifestyle. Besides following the Non-Diet way of eating, exercise is one of the best things you can do to avoid stroke.

When you exercise, your heart beats more rapidly, your arteries widen to provide more oxygen, your arterial blood flow improves and glucose and cholesterol levels decrease. Exercise also generates new stem cells that repair brain and heart cells and build new blood vessels, and it even grows new brain cells, a process called neurogenesis.

The most common risk factors for stroke are hypertension, diabetes, high cholesterol and obesity. Smoking elevates levels of CRP that damage blood vessels in the brain. Uncontrolled high blood pressure also damages arteries, yet two-thirds of Americans diagnosed with hypertension do not have their blood pressure under control.

Most people don't think about how their lifestyle and diet impact the brain until it's too late. Your brain's rate of aging depends on your family history, but lifestyle choices and environmental exposures make the biggest difference. The "disease-fighting" nutrients offered in the Non-Diet program can lower all the risk factors of stroke and help prevent memory decline and Alzheimer's disease. The earlier you start, the sooner you'll reap the benefits and protect your amazing brain from the devastating complications of vascular disease.

Chapter 7

"Female-pattern" Vascular Disease

More than half of my neurosurgery patients require a cardiac clearance before I can perform surgery. Any symptoms such as shortness of breath or chest discomfort, and conditions such as obesity and diabetes require a thorough workup before the anesthesiologist will consent to put my patient to sleep. If the electrocardiogram (EKG), echocardiogram, chest X-ray or blood test is abnormal, surgery may be postponed or even cancelled. We can't afford complications related to vascular disease, and neither can you. The first symptom in 50 percent of the people with heart disease is *death*.

And so begins my recollection of an event that happened several years ago. Sara, a 39-year-old woman, came to my clinic complaining of right-sided flank pain. She was very fit and robust, a former college volleyball player who had become a well-respected engineer in the field of water conservancy. Her doctor had recommended a course of powerful pain-killers, and that's why she came to see me. She knew that I rarely prescribed addicting medications.

I performed a neurological exam but nothing seemed amiss. Routine X-ray and MRI were negative. I was perplexed about the source of her pain, but I decided to air on the side of conservancy and referred her to an internist in the clinic across the street.

It was lunch time. By coincidence, Sara and I walked out of my office together. It was humid and breezy, and I noticed a few storm clouds on the horizon. I still remember every single unsettling second of what happened next. Sara dropped on the tarmac. She fell just beyond the walkway leading to the hospital and clinic buildings. Her face and neck flushed a bright red as sweat came pouring out of every body orifice. As I kneeled down on the ground beside her to begin emergency CPR, she suddenly threw her head back and balled her fists with a startling force. For a split-second, my mind flashed back to the moment when my first wife had given the final, all-encompassing push and my first son was born.

I shouted out Sara's name as I thrust my hands together on top of her chest and began compressions—*one one-thousand, two one-thousand* ... I also shouted to the medical staff coming and going to call 911. The emergency department and all its life-saving technology were less than

500 feet away. I continued my compressions, then felt for Sara's carotid artery but it was still. Her face had gone from bright red, to deep purple, to ashen and gray. A pool of sweat spread-out beneath us. I continued CPR until the emergency medical staff arrived, but knew that Sara would die without immediate intervention.

Sara's near-death would change the way I view women and heart disease. More than half of all Americans who die of vascular disease succumb suddenly without warning. The other half have the disease lurking in their bodies for many years before it strikes. For women, angina—a sign of advanced heart disease—may feel like nausea, shortness of breath, or even a radiating pain in the jaw or back. Any pain between the ears and navel—left *or* right side—is suspect in a woman.

Medical schools once taught that women were at lower risk for heart disease than men, but today we know that more women than men die each year of heart disease.[50] Over 250,000 women die from heart disease in the United State each year—that's more than the 14 leading causes of death *combined*. Still, heart disease isn't a standard part of a woman's annual health care assessment. As a result, women are often misdiagnosed or never diagnosed. A woman's first heart attack is more often fatal than a man's. Women are also less likely to survive bypass surgery, and more likely to suffer severe symptoms of heart failure. Women tend to experience symptoms of heart disease years later than men, but even that scenario has exceptions, as in the case of Sara, or as in the case of my 40 year old daughter and the co-author of this book, Kim.

Vascular disease is dynamic, unpredictable, and most of all an equal opportunity killer. Even with the recent surge in research, heart disease is poorly understood in women, from the expression of the symptoms all the way down to some of the basic mechanisms that cause the disease. For my daughter, the problems lie not in the coronary arteries, but in the smaller branches and tiny capillaries that nourish the heart muscle, pathology referred to as "coronary microvascular disease." After a close call during her third pregnancy, Kim sought a second opinion from Carl Pepine, M.D., a renowned cardiologist and researcher who focuses on women with heart disease. Tiny clogged vessels don't show up on standard diagnostic tests, so doctors assume that something other than heart disease may be causing symptoms such as back or shoulder pain, fatigue, light-headedness or chest pain. The way to diagnose small vessel disease is through an endothelial dysfunction test, a special type of coronary angiogram involving a Doppler wire threaded inside a coronary artery to measure blood flow. The procedure uses the same diagnostic technique that interventional cardiologists use on a regular basis before inserting a balloon or stent in a blocked artery.

About 3 million American men and women have been diagnosed with coronary microvascular disease, although the percentage of men is much smaller. Another 2-3 million men and women have the disease but haven't been properly diagnosed, according to estimates by Noel Bairy Merz, M.D. This puts them at risk for heart attack, stroke and heart failure. Dr. Bairy Merz is a professor at the medical school at the University of California, Los Angeles, and the chair of the National Institutes of Health (NIH)-sponsored WISE (Women's Ischemic Syndrome Evaluation) initiative, which is investigating potential methods for more effective diagnosis and evaluation of coronary artery disease in women. She recommends additional testing for people with coronary artery disease symptoms and no evidence of clogged arteries on a coronary angiogram—the diagnostic tool for visualizing narrowing or blockage in the large coronary arteries. Dr. Bairy Merz believes nutrition plays one of the largest roles in the development and progression of vascular disease.

Women as Caregivers

Society socializes women to be nurturers and caregivers, a behavior that extends to their husbands, parents and children, but often not to themselves. "We have to overcome that psychology of women that they want to take care of everybody else in the family, and they take care of themselves last," said Steve Nissen, M.D., the Chairman of the Department of Cardiovascular Medicine at the Cleveland Clinic.

Physically, a woman's heart is no different from a man's heart, but the spectrum of vascular disease presents differently in women. Instead of one main blockage, arteries in many women go into spasm or have diffuse buildup *inside* the walls of the arteries, which can be easily missed on angiogram but is just as dangerous. According to experts such as Dr. Pepine, women's bodies remodel their arteries to accommodate the plaque, just as women remodel their arteries to accommodate blood flow when they are pregnant. Peanut butter spread thickly inside the wall of the artery is another way to think about the presentation of "female-pattern" vascular disease.

Vascular disease is the number one killer of women. Although rates of coronary artery disease have declined in men, they haven't declined as rapidly in women. Research and population studies show that vascular disease affects men and women equally. Yet when they are asked to identify the greatest threat to their health, most American women name breast cancer, a popular misconception in part due to the tremendous campaign efforts to fund research for the cancer. Vascular disease kills far more women than breast cancer, but there's still no yearly equivalent to the mammogram. And knowledge about prevention and treatment of the disease in women continues to lag behind research about men. In 1991, the National Institutes for Health commissioned the Women's Health Initiative, one of the largest prevention studies in U.S. history, to address the gap.

One of the biggest and most controversial findings of the landmark study was that hormone therapy had serious risks, and did not prevent vascular disease in postmenopausal women. Researchers found that when estrogen is combined with progestin, the way women have to take it after menopause, there is an increased risk of breast cancer, blood clots and stroke.[51] They also discovered that the risk of heart attack increases for women taking estrogen therapy over the age of 60. Another study on women who took birth control pills found they had three times the normal levels of an enzyme linked with vascular inflammation. The lesson behind these findings is that medicine is an enterprise of constantly changing knowledge, uncertain information, and fallible professionals. Natural remedies have much fewer risks.

A report in the *Annals of Internal Medicine* found that doctors often fail to prescribe even the most basic preventive strategies for women, such as taking statins to lower cholesterol or aspirin to lower the risk of stroke.[52] Sudden death is the first evidence of vascular disease in half of its victims. "Early detection, accurate diagnosis and proper treatment" of vascular disease are the keys to a better outcome, according to WomenHeart, a patient advocacy group for women with vascular disease. For their own sake, and for the sake of those who love them, women have to become "informed advocates" in their pursuit of the best vascular care.

The new focus on women and vascular disease is an opportunity for women to reassess what's for dinner, and how their choices not only affect the health of their loved ones, but their own lives too.

PART III:
GET TO KNOW AND DEAL
WITH YOUR RISK FACTORS

Chapter 8

The Cause and Effect of Chronic Inflammation

The best marker for inflammation, and the most consistent marker of poor vascular prognosis is CRP, short for C-reactive protein. CRP helps measure systemic inflammation, the level of inflammation in our body, and the overall health of our arteries. During acute inflammation, the liver produces higher levels of CRP and releases it into the blood stream. Higher levels of CRP are common in people with inflammatory disease, but can also help predict impending coronary events.

The higher your CRP level, the more at risk you may be for vascular disease or heart attack and stroke, even if your other indicators look normal. People with higher CRP have three times the risk for heart attack, stroke and restenosis of coronary arteries after angioplasty. Elevated CRP levels also predict recurrent coronary events in patients with unstable angina. Ask your doctor to order a high-sensitivity CRP test to get some idea of your risk.

Measuring Homocysteine

A few years ago, homocysteine, a by-product of amino acid metabolism, was thought to be one of the key explanations for otherwise unexplained heart attacks and strokes. But more recent studies have been inconclusive. The American Heart Association (AHA) does not yet consider homocysteine a major risk factor for heart disease. However, you may want to ask your doctor to check your homocysteine level if you have a family history of premature vascular disease, or suffer an unexplained heart attack or stroke. Many doctors screen for homocysteine when diagnosing vascular disease.

Your body uses homocysteine to make protein, and to build and maintain tissue. In excess levels, homocysteine may irritate or even damage arteries, triggering low-grade inflammation and elevating the risk of clotting. Genetic defects or diet, specifically deficiencies in the folates (folic acid, Vitamins B6 and B12), can raise homocysteine levels. Eating plenty of citrus fruits, grains, lentils, chickpeas and green, leafy vegetables is the safest and most effective way to get folic acid and reduce homocysteine.

Up to 40 percent of people with vascular disease have high homocysteine levels. Attempts to inhibit homocysteine with supplements have not been effective in reducing the risk of vascular events in these patients, according to a comprehensive study published in the *Journal of the American Medical Association*. But because some studies correlate elevated homocysteine with more severe coronary artery disease, many experts, including the doctors at the Mayo and Cleveland Clinics, recommend screening for homocysteine to help determine the state of a patient's vascular health.

Fibrinogen and Blood Clotting

Fibrinogen, a protein produced by the liver that signals our body to form blood clots, may help doctors determine vascular risk in patients with normal lipid profiles. Elevated fibrinogen may damage blood vessel walls or promote inflammation and excessive clumping of platelets, the type of blood cell responsible for clotting. Acute thrombosis, the sudden formation of a blood clot at the site of an atherosclerotic plaque, is responsible for 95 percent of all vascular events.

Heavy drinking, smoking and inactivity can raise fibrinogen; exercise can lower it, according to the Women's Health Study.[53] Your doctor may check your fibrinogen level if you are on estrogen or have an increased risk of vascular disease, heart attack or stroke.

The Powerful Omegas

Omega fatty acids are essential (ESFs) and must be obtained from the food we eat. The saturated fat in meat and dairy products is a direct source of arachidonic acid, an omega-6 fatty acid. Loading up on high-fat meats such as hamburger or prime rib, promotes the buildup of arachidonic acid in bodily tissues, boosting inflammatory prostaglandin production. Conversely, consuming a diet with higher levels of omega-3 tends to reduce the level of arachidonic acid and the production of numerous inflammatory leukotrienes in our bodies' tissues.

We tend to associate omega-3 fatty acids with fish oil, but fish get the acids from green algae. Seeds contain more of another essential fatty acid: omega-6. The two omegas perform very different functions. Omega-3s play an important role in our neurological development, the metabolism of glucose, the permeability of cell walls, as well as the reduction of inflammation. Omega-6s are involved in the rigidity of our cell walls, fat storage, blood clotting and immune response.

Manufacturers market a large variety of omega-3 dietary supplements and promote the fats in everything from tortillas to baby formula. Fish cooked in canola, flaxseed or walnut oil may be a good way to lower the risk of dementia, according to a recent study published in the journal Neurology. The four-year study found that those who regularly consumed omega-3-rich oils reduced their risk of dementia by 60 percent, compared to those didn't. Eating fruits and vegetables was associated with a similar dip in risk.[54]

How Much Fish Oil?

Fish oil may fend off a variety of ailments. Eating a one-half gram supplement, or salmon twice weekly may be enough if you are healthy.

The American Heart Association recommends that heart patients take a one-gram supplement or more each day.

Consuming omega-3s from eating two servings of fish weekly, improves vascular health by decreasing inflammation and triglyceride levels, lowering blood pressure, and decreasing the risk of arrhythmias. The antithrombotic properties of omega-3s also reduce the risk of blood clots—the number one cause of heart attack and stroke.[55]

While some omega-6 fatty acids are essential for our health, consuming too much in our diet may make vascular inflammation worse. Omega-6s are found in egg yolks, poultry, cereals, vegetable oils, baked goods and margarine. Omega-6s support skin health and help make our blood "sticky" so it is able to clot. But when the omega-6s aren't balanced with sufficient amounts of omega-3s, problems can ensue.

Omega-6 fatty acids produce inflammatory eicosanoids that promote pain, signal blood platelets to clot, and depress brain function. They have a powerful effect on triglycerides, blood pressure, systemic inflammation and the development or progression of vascular disease, including the occurrence of sudden cardiac death, heart attack or stroke. Linoleic acid is the most prevalent omega-6 in our SAD diet of processed foods, red meat, dairy products and eggs. Over 60 years ago, the American dietary ratio of omega-6 to omega-3 was 1 to 2. Today, the ratio is 25 to 1. Bad fats compete with good fats, so it's important to minimize the intake of saturated fats while consuming enough good fats.[56]

Consuming complex carbohydrates such as fresh fruits, vegetables, whole grains and legumes disable free radicals, the primary mechanisms in inflammation. Losing weight means fewer cytokines, the inflammatory molecules. No smoking, moderate alcohol intake and most of all—regular exercise, 30 minutes a day most days of the week, also reduce inflammation levels. Even flossing your teeth combats chronic inflammation. If you want to stop inflammationin yourself and your family members, take action. It's never too late too reverse the collateral damage.

CHAPTER 9

CHOLESTEROL: THE MAD PAINTER OF ARTERIES

Cholesterol is one of the most profoundly important vascular markers, but inflammation ranks higher in terms of immediate risk—you can have a normal lipid profile but high levels of CRP, escalating the threat of heart attack and stroke. Beginning as early as grade school, excess cholesterol from your diet lays the foundation for plaque. Later in life, high cholesterol levels strongly correlate with vascular disease and death.

Americans are doing better at controlling cholesterol through diet and drugs. And the recent widespread elimination of trans fats from processed foods will help. But more than 100 million Americans still have total blood cholesterol values of 200 and higher. Of these, about 40 million American adults have levels of 240 or above.[57] Research from the National Heart, Lung and Blood Institute's (NHLB) Framingham Study, the ongoing study of vascular disease in Framingham, Massachusetts, has found that the risk of fatal heart attack rises gradually at a cholesterol level of 150 milligrams per deciliter of blood serum, accelerates at the level of 200, and shoots for the sky at 230.

Cholesterol is a soft, waxy substance that paints the wall of every living cell, as well as fulfills vital chemical functions. We don't need to consume cholesterol. The body produces it to build cells and make vitamins and hormones, including vitamin D and all substances of steroids in our body, such as cortisol, progesterone and estrogen. Enzymes synthesize cholesterol and other fatty acids in the liver from acetic acid, an insoluble substance that manufacturers reproduce for a broad range of chemical products from vinegar and preservatives, to its highly concentrated form in plastics, rubber and insecticides.

A diet high in saturated fats from consuming meat, eggs and dairy products can raise blood cholesterol levels to the degree that cholesterol invades the walls of coronary arteries, reducing critical nutrients and blood flow to the heart. For every one percent *increase* in the amount of cholesterol in the blood, there is about a two percent increase in the risk of heart attack or stroke. Conversely, every one percent *reduction* from the average cholesterol level reduces the risk by about two percent. Medicine typically subdivides cholesterol into two types: low-density lipoprotein (LDL) and high-density lipoprotein (HDL).

LDL, the "Lousy" Cholesterol

One of the most important fatty acids in the body is LDL, the "bad" cholesterol. Cholesterol is insoluble in blood and must combine with fat and protein molecules in order to be transported into cells. The combination, lipoprotein, transports cholesterol throughout the body like a fleet of railroad cars. LDL transports about 60 to 80 percent of the body's cholesterol. Cells throughout the body absorb LDL as building blocks for hormones and other vital life substances. How and where the body transports LDL, and in what amount, determines whether or not LDL becomes harmful.

LDL and very low-density lipoprotein are tiny lipids. As lipids circulate throughout the blood vessels, they encounter twists and turns, and changes in pressure that can force them inside the artery wall, triggering the body's immune response. As we discussed in the chapter on inflammation, white blood cells flock to the site to ingest the lipoproteins, expanding the elastic wall with the foam of their engorged plaque, and promoting the cycle of vascular inflammation.

LDL is a more accurate marker of cardiac risk than cholesterol alone. The goal in current federal guidelines is to get LDL below 100, but we recommend levels even lower. You should keep your LDL under 80 if you have no vascular disease, and 70 if you do have the disease. Lowering LDL is far more effective than coronary angioplasty, stenting or bypass surgery because it reduces plaque and vascular inflammation, the heart of the disease process. Treating high cholesterol reduces the short-term risk of heart attack and stroke by as much as 40 percent in patients with vascular disease. Following a Non-Dieting way of life and using statin drug therapy, if needed, can reduce LDL a great deal. A *total* cholesterol level at 150 or below will make you "heart-attack proof."

Diet and Cholesterol

The discovery in 1912 that dietary cholesterol generates atherosclerosis, turned attention to the perils of fat and cholesterol, eclipsing research on dietary protein. We don't hear a lot about the dangers of animal protein, and that is a big mistake. Consuming animal-based proteins such as meat, eggs and dairy can increase blood cholesterol levels. The Oxford-Cornell China Project found that animal protein was one of the biggest elevators of LDL. Dr. Esselstyn, of the Cleveland

Clinic, tells his patients if you want to lower your cholesterol: "Don't eat anything that has a mother or a face (no meat, poultry or fish)."[58]

Dr. Esselstyn also stipulates that patients cannot consume oil of any kind, including "heart healthy" olive oil which contains high levels of artery-clogging saturated fat, the same fat in meat. Fully 25 percent of the subjects in the Lyon Diet Heart Study who consumed a Mediterranean-style diet—which allows such oils—had experienced a heart attack, stroke or died of vascular complications. Several studies support the directive to stop using oils of any kind if you want to reverse or prevent vascular disease.

Saturated fat and dietary cholesterol found in baked goods and fried foods also raise blood cholesterol, although animal proteins affect it at a much higher rate. Cholesterol is only found in animals. Plant-based foods contain no cholesterol. If you reduce your daily intake of animal products such as meat and dairy, and increase your intake of complex-carbohydrates—vegetables, whole grains, legumes and fruit—you will lower your blood cholesterol level, as well as lose weight and feel better.

In Colin T. Campbell's China Study, the average animal protein intake of the Chinese was 7.1 grams per day (about the equivalent of three chicken nuggets), whereas the average American intake was a whopping 70 grams of animal protein per day (about the equivalent of 30 chicken nuggets). Eating saturated fat and animal protein increases the amount of cholesterol and fats in the body. Is it any wonder that vascular disease is the leadingcause of death in a country where the cheeseburger is the most popular restaurant meal?

HDL, the "Healthy" Cholesterol

What about HDL cholesterol? HDL, the "good" cholesterol is also made of protein but very low fat, which produces a dense, stable package that doesn't unravel easily when it hits the interior wall of an artery. HDL assists in undoing the damage brought on by LDL—it's a scavenger that works to remove LDL cholesterol from the arteries and delivers it to the liver for disposal. You need more HDL to counter increases in LDL. HDL is about 25 percent of total cholesterol.

The average woman fares better than the average man. Female sex hormones such as progesterone raise HDL cholesterol. A score of 60 will put you in the low-risk category, but many doctors only target 40 for men and 50 for women. Smoking, obesity and inactivity lower HDL cholesterol. You can raise and keep your HDL high by exercising, losing weight and, most of all, avoiding saturated fat and consuming a high fiber diet of fruit and vegetables. HDL and triglycerides tend to go in opposite directions—a high triglyceride level often means you'll have a low HDL level.

Triglycerides

Checking your blood serum triglyceride level is another important cardiac marker to assess your risk for vascular disease. Your body converts unused calories into triglycerides and stores them in fat cells. Hormones regulate the release of triglycerides from fatty tissues to meet the body's needs for energy between meals. A small amount of triglycerides is found in the bloodstream as lipoproteins. Elevated triglyceride levels often correlate with vascular complications, especially in patients who are obese, hypertensive or diabetic. A normal level of triglycerides is 50 to 150. Inactivity, alcohol, smoking, skipping meals or eating large portions of foods all at once can raise triglycerides.

Triglycerides respond quickly to diet and lifestyle changes. Omega-3s are very effective in reducing triglycerides. A review of fish oil and vascular disease found that taking 2,000 milligrams of fish oil daily lowered triglycerides by 25 percent in healthy people, and by 40-50 percent in people with high triglyceride levels.[59] Specific medications can help lower triglycerides if lifestyle changes and supplements alone don't help.

Know Your Numbers

Reducing total cholesterol, especially LDL, is one of the best strategies to avoid suffering a heart attack or stroke. If you have a family history of heart disease, ask your doctor to run a lipid profile—no matter what your age. About five percent of Americans have a rare genetic disorder called "familial hypercholesterolemia," where the body cannot properly metabolize cholesterol. The disorder can lead to premature heart disease, heart attacks and strokes. Check your cholesterol levels early in life when it matters most, so that you can do something about it. Your doctor may conclude a level of 180 or more is fine, but I believe 150 will make you heart-attack proof. The frequency of vascular events drops two to three percent for every one percent drop in cholesterol.[60]

Chapter 10
Weight: the Wages of Cheesecake

Take off your clothes and stand in front of a mirror. What do you see? Whatever you see, take a pledge right now to love your body. Bodies come in all shapes and sizes, and some of us, especially women, are more susceptible to weight gain. The goal of this chapter isn't to scare anyone into losing weight, rather to make people aware of the serious health risks related to obesity. Fat can be toxic, spewing out substances that contribute to hypertension, insulin resistance, diabetes, dyslipidemia, depression, vascular disease and other illnesses, including the cancers listed on pages 37 or page 145. The illnesses may not be perceptible today. As the eminent surgeon and nutritionist Caldwell Esselstyn, Jr., M.D. noted, "Sometimes it takes decades of self-imposed damage before symptoms develop."

Fat and Getting Fatter

Over the past decade, we've had a mind-boggling increase in what is fast emerging as the most serious and costly health problem in the U.S.: morbid obesity. About 35 percent, or 72 million, American adults are obese. And of that number, 7 million adults are morbidly obese, a health condition which substantially raises the risk of mortality (death) and morbidity (chronic disease). The rate of obesity has increased by almost 25 percent, but the rate of morbid obesity has grown even faster: people with a Body Mass Index (BMI) over 40 increased by 50 percent.

Perhaps most alarmingly, people with a BMI over 50, extreme obesity, grew by 75 percent, *three times faster* than the rate of obesity. Our children are not immune from the epidemic. We've seen a 300 percent

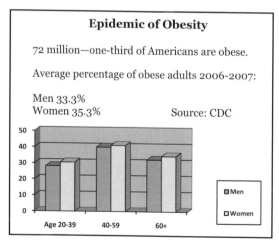

Epidemic of Obesity

72 million—one-third of Americans are obese.

Average percentage of obese adults 2006-2007:

Men 33.3%
Women 35.3%   Source: CDC

Age 20-39   40-59   60+

☐ Men
☐ Women

increase in overweight children. Obesity conditions are the fastest growing cause of death, and the second leading cause of preventable death. New research based on U.S. and Chinese population studies found the lowest rates of death in persons who were of normal weight.[61]

Retrofitting the Overweight

A recent press release from the *American College of Radiology* described how Joel Pond, a veterinary technician at Chicago's Lincoln Park Zoo, routinely fields calls from radiologists and other physicians looking for super-sized scanners for their obese patients.[62] Medicine can't keep up with the rising number of super-sized patients. Ambulances, gurneys, wheelchairs and hospital beds are just some of the medical equipment that has been retrofitted to meet the needs of obese patients.

Although the term "obesity" describes someone 100 or more pounds overweight, many of the patients that my partners and I see tip the scales at 400, 500 or more pounds. Our national statistics support what I see on a regular basis in our clinic. My 40-year-old patient, Paul, was 5'10" and weighed about 440 pounds when he arrived at the Emergency Room complaining of nausea and a severe headache.

Paul's BMI was a massive 63. A thin film of sweat covered his face and neck. I could tell he was in a lot of pain. We had to order a giant cart to transfer him from the ER to the surgical theater where I would operate on a bulging cerebral aneurysm in his brain. It took six people doing backbreaking work to lift him onto the two operating tables that we had to tie together.

Paul had been an active, sociable and bright young man of normal weight until he was struck down by meningitis at age 23. He remained comatose for two weeks and was fed by a gastric feeding tube. When he finally awoke, he recalled feeing extremely hungry and frustrated because no one could understand his requests for more food. As his voice improved, his needs were met. But following his illness, his anxiety about food persisted. He had an enormous appetite and ate constantly. Within a year, he gained 100 pounds. Ultimately, his obsession for food led to extreme obesity and disability. He was unable to work and spent all of his time watching TV or playing video games. He rarely left his house because he could barely walk. Hunger is a learned behavior. Early experiences with food often drive later disturbances in eating.

Searching for a Cause

Scientists are trying to find the cause of the obesity epidemic beyond the obvious: too many people are eating too much for their metabolic rate. Morbidly obese people do not gain weight like people of normal weight—it's not just an issue of willpower or personal responsibility. Abnormal metabolism, brain chemistry, addiction, psychology and genetic mutations are just some of the reasons why the cause of morbid obesity is not as obvious as it may seem, and why it's one of the biggest mysteries of medicine.

When Yankee Stadium was renovated in 1974, about 50 years after its construction in the 1920s, workers had to reduce the number of seats to offer wider seats to accommodate the increase in overweight fans. Pre-World War II, fatal heart attacks were virtually unheard of, and very few people were obese. Today, 65 percent of Americans are overweight or obese. Why has America gotten so fat?

One, we've become sedentary. Neighborhoods are spread out and often lack sidewalks, but are never far away from an omnipresent 7-11, McDonald's or Pizza Hut. The Internet, television, iPods, cell phones and other hand-held devices allow us to be passive consumers of entertainment and sports, versus active producers. We also sit behind a desk all day, while our grandparents expended energy working. Automobiles have replaced walking. Even the mailman used to walk. Those who must work long hours to pay the rent have very little leisure time and often cannot afford expensive gym or elite club memberships.

Two, American technological innovations in food production and transportation have reduced the cost of processed foods, making high sugar, high fat, "energy dense" food cheap and readily available. American families are consuming more food and 800 more calories per family member, per day than their relatives did in the late 1950s. Part of the problem is the surge in sugars and fat in our SAD, each has increased over 20 percent since 1977.[63] Much of the increase in sugar is due to our soft drink consumption. A 42-ounce Coke, available for as little as 89 cents at McDonald's, contains about 400 calories and 40 teaspoons of sugar. The average size of a soft drink in 1955, the year that McDonald's opened, was 7 ounces. Taste, cost and convenience, not health, drive the majority of our food choices.

Some Lower Energy-Dense Foods		
Food	% water	Calories/100 g
Navel Orange	85.97	49
Red Grapes	80.54	69
Watermelon	91.45	30
Iceberg Lettuce	95.07	15
Vidalia Onion	91.24	32
Green Pepper (sweet, green)	93.89	20
Watercress	95.11	11
Spinach	91.40	23

Figure 4: Lower energy-dense foods. These foods are high in fiber and water content and low in calories. Lower energy-dense foods are also good sources of vitamins and cancer-fighting ingredients such as antioxidants. (Source: USDA)

Falling Food Prices, Expanding Families

Today food takes up only 10 percent of the average household spending. According to the USDA, 100 years ago, food took up almost 25 percent of the family budget. Harvard economics professor, David M. Cutler, noted the chief economic reasons for the rise of the obesity epidemic over the past 50 years: the price of food fell, the cost of preparing foods fell, energy needs for work and home fell, and the value of women's time rose:

> Technological innovations—including vacuum packing, improved preservatives, deep freezing, artificial flavors, and microwaves—have enabled food manufacturers to cook food centrally and ship it to consumers for rapid consumption. In 1965, a married woman who didn't work spent over two hours per day cooking and cleaning up from meals. In 1995, the same tasks took less than half the time.[64]

Over 75 percent of the planet doesn't have high rates of obesity or vascular disease because their traditional plant-based diet doesn't put them at risk. Our market-driven economy, advancing technology, SAD diet and ancient genes have collided in such a way as to create a lethal environment for our health. Western nations have replaced malnutrition and infectious disease with the epidemic of obesity. We are in the middle of a health crisis that may have profound health effects for decades still to come. Unlike a viral epidemic with natural enemies, the obesity epidemic has powerful allies in the industrial food chain to keep it going all the way to the graveyard. People who are obese have a 50 to 100 percent increased risk of premature death from *all* causes, according to the U.S. Department of Health and Human Services. Sadly, our children will suffer the most.

Obesity, even in children, is an independent risk factor for vascular disease. Today adolescents and teens, in particular, are eating large amounts of high-caloric, artery-clogging fast food. Restaurant food makes up 50 percent of the meals families eat in a year. The saturated fat in these rich foods doesn't satiate us as quickly as fiber-rich whole foods, which means we may end up eating larger portions to feel full. Consuming too many calories puts the body into a state of oxidative stress—the body cannot use all the extra fuel. And because the liver cannot break down the extra load, blood sugars, blood fats and blood pressure all increase, adding fuel to the fire of vascular inflammation.

An increasing amount of scientific evidence points to obesity as an inflammatory condition. For years, doctors and scientists were aware of a relationship between obesity, insulin resistance, and vascular disease, but they couldn't pinpoint a mechanistic link. New research suggests that abdominal fat may be the culprit.

Weight-related Conditions
- Acid-reflux, heartburn
- Asthma, respiratory problems
- Back pain, disc herniation
- Cancer: endometrial, breast, ovarian, prostate, colon
- Coronary artery and microvascular disease, angina, stroke, heart attack, sudden death, heart failure
- Depression, eating disorders
- Erectile dysfunction
- Gallbladder disease, gallstones
- Gout
- Dyslipidemia
- Hypertension
- Insomnia, sleep apnea
- Insulin resistance, metabolic syndrome, and Type 2 diabetes
- Osteoarthritis

Belly Fat, the Unofficial Organ

We used to think that fat was benign, just a despised consequence of cheeseburgers and French fries. Within the past three decades of our ever increasing waistlines, the scientific view of belly fat has evolved from a storage bin for excess calories, to a dynamic *organ* called the "omentum" which releases hormones and inflammatory substances into our bloodstream. These bioactive substances affect metabolism and weight, and promote the risks of many illnesses linked to vascular disease. Today doctors and researchers believe that obesity and waist circumference are two of the most powerful predictors of mortality. People with an apple versus a pear shape face higher risks of heart attack, stroke and diabetes.

Our biological destiny is to store fat. The omentum, an apron-like web of fat that hangs down in front of our large intestine, evolved as a fat depot to support our ancestors during periods of famine. Thousands of years ago, "thrifty genes" were also necessary for our ancestors' survival when they had to hunt and forage for food and didn't know when they were going to eat again. Thrifty genes improve our natural energy stores by retaining weight in the omentum, buttocks and hips, but have become a liability today. When we're under stress and overeat, the omentum is the first place we gain weight. Conversely, belly fat is the first place we lose weight.

In most parts of the body, fat is just under the skin (subcutaneous) or over the muscle. But the omentum, which comprises about one-third of our visceral fat, is packed deeply between and around organs, and generates more metabolic activity than the fat on our behinds. Some doctors refer to the omentum as a tumor because it generates so many hormones and chemicals, some of them toxic to the surrounding organs. For instance, the liver metabolizes visceral fat and turns it into fatty molecules of cholesterol (lipids) that circulate in the blood and collect on the walls of arteries, forming plaques.

Fat Fact
Each year about 400,000 Americans die of obesity-related conditions, primarily vacular disease

The total number of fat cells in our bodies remains the same throughout adulthood. Losing or gaining weight affects only the *amount* of fat stored in the cells, not the number of cells. Fat cells can increase over 1,000 times in size. The larger the fat cells in the omentum, the greater the risk will be for insulin resistance. Obese people have huge fat cells with 50 to 75 percent more mass than fat cells in thin people. The pancreas has to keep making extra insulin to overcome the resistance of these larger cells. The obesity epidemic is responsible for the diabetes epidemic, as obese people literally outgrow the capacity of their pancreas.

Because of the link to insulin resistance and inflammation, abdominal obesity increases the risk of vascular disease by 300 percent. Research from the Framingham Heart Study found that abdominal girth was an independent risk factor for stroke and heart attack, even in the absence of high blood pressure or diabetes.[65] Inflammation plays a major part in the connection between obesity and sudden death from vascular disease. A cardiologist once told me that men with beer bellies were "walking heart attacks." Even a skinny person who has a large belly faces a higher risk of vascular complications. If you're male with a waist size of more than 40 inches, or a female with more than a 35-inch waist, ask your doctor to check the level of inflammation in your body with an inexpensive CRP blood test (see Chapter 1 for more information on CRP).

The Leptin Link to Body-Weight Regulation

Leptin is a powerful hormone released by visceral fat cells in the omentum, buttocks and hips to regulate key brain chemicals related to obesity. Researchers at Dundee University in Scotland discovered a link between leptin and the brain's frontal cortex, the executive center for decision-making, learning and memory. Leptin has a profound influence on our brain and body, affecting eating behavior and metabolism.

Fat cells generate leptin to communicate with the hypothalamus, the gland in the brain that controls appetite. Leptin "tells" the brain how much fat the body has so that the brain can adjust eating and metabolism to keep fat stores at a certain level. If enough fat is in storage, the hypothalamus signals the adrenal gland to increase the metabolic rate. As we gain weight, our expanding fat layers make more and more leptin, which signals the brain to quiet our appetite in an attempt to stop the accumulating fat. When leptin levels are too low, our appetite becomes ravenous, and that's why crash diets don't work. Leptin levels drop after a crash diet, which increases the appetite and slows metabolism. If leptin levels fall dramatically, we may get a big rebound of appetite and gain even more weight.

Leptin regulates food intake, storage and metabolism throughout the body, but the leptin balance of people who are obese changes over time. Because fat cells make leptin, an obese person has a much higher level of the powerful hormone circulating in their body, but they develop a resistance to it, which may explain why the obese often cannot control their appetites or feel satiated after eating. Obesity is a vicious cycle.

Another important hormone generated by fat is adiponectin, a substance that increases sensitivity to insulin. When people become obese, their fat cells make less adiponectin, increasing the risk of both diabetes and vascular disease.

Scientists have identified at least 15 other major biochemicals released by visceral fat cells, including important inflammatory molecules called interleukin-6 (IL-6) and tumor necrosis factor (TNF). When metabolism is skewed by obesity, these immune substances that normally aid us, backfire, and can actually increase CRP and cancerous cells, as well as vascular disease, Alzheimer's and other inflammatory illnesses. The Harvard School of Public Health found that obesity raises the risk for one-third of all cancers, including the most common: lung, breast, and colon.[66] From a clinical perspective, obesity influences a remarkably broad spectrum of health complications related to inflammation.

Living Large

Beyond all the physical health risks, the emotional pain of being obese, the social isolation of "wearing" a condition that most everyone believes to be within your control, is a heavy burden to bear. In our society's obsession with physical beauty, we have created an environment so hostile to the idea of obesity, that overweight people have become marginalized. They may even fail to show up for routine medical appointments because they don't want to be badgered about their weight by their doctors.

The same biochemicals that regulate our emotions, e.g., serotonin, norepinephrine and dopamine, are active in the hypothalamus, the part of the brain that influences eating and satiety. Many people who are depressed lose their appetite or turn to food for comfort, and some may even binge to "medicate" their feelings. When we eat chocolate, our body releases trace amounts of biochemicals associated with well-being and alertness. Similar to the biochemistry of drug addiction, indulging in foods like chocolate to excess can reduce the number of "receptors" in the brain for these happy biochemicals and lead to a cycle of compulsive overeating, leading to obesity. Following the advice in Chapter 11 and the Non-Diet approach to food are the two most effective ways to break-free of food addictions.

If you're obese and lose as little as five to 10 percent of your weight, you can dramatically reduce your health risks, especially the risks related to vascular disease. Barring bariatric surgery, a high-risk procedure that costs $25 to $50,000, the only way to lose weight is to ensure that energy in (calories consumed) is less than energy out (calories expended).

The weight-loss industry and media are guilty of promoting trendy, potentially harmful diets, even though several studies from our leading academic institutions have proven diets don't work. The human body has a biological "set point" that adjusts our metabolic rate up or down whenever we gain or lose weight. For example, a healthy woman with a set point of 140 pounds is unlikely to shed or gain more than 20 pounds. When we take in too many calories and gain weight, our set point kicks-in and metabolism speeds up to process the excess calories and lose the weight. But if we continue to take in more calories than we burn, our metabolic resistance loses strength and our body reestablishes its set point to a new, higher weight.

If you want to burn up excess fat and keep it off, you have to speed up your metabolism through aerobic exercise and by eating frequent, small meals of starchy fruits and vegetables, legumes and whole grains. Complex carbohydrates are nature's fat burners, a topic we discuss in Chapter 12. When you lose weight slowly, your metabolism shifts to a new set point for that weight. Extreme dieting and deprivation, in the long run, only generate an endless cycle of weight loss, overindulgence, and gaining weight back again. Following the secrets of the Non-Diet will be one of the most powerful weapons you have against obesity.

Body Mass Index (BMI) Table
BMI Categories:
  Underweight = <18.5
  Normal weight = 18.5-24.9
  Overweight = 25-29.9
  Obesity = BMI of 30 or greater

BMI	19	20	21	22	23	24	25	26	27	28	29	30	31	32	33	34	35
Height (inches)							Body Weight (pounds)										
58	91	96	100	105	110	115	119	124	129	134	138	143	148	153	158	162	167
59	94	99	104	109	114	119	124	128	133	138	143	148	153	158	163	168	173
60	97	102	107	112	118	123	128	133	138	143	148	153	158	163	168	174	179
61	100	106	111	116	122	127	132	137	143	148	153	158	164	169	174	180	185
62	104	109	115	120	126	131	136	142	147	153	158	164	169	175	180	186	191
63	107	113	118	124	130	135	141	146	152	158	163	169	175	180	186	191	197
64	110	116	122	128	134	140	145	151	157	163	169	174	180	186	192	197	204
65	114	120	126	132	138	144	150	156	162	168	174	180	186	192	198	204	210
66	118	124	130	136	142	148	155	161	167	173	179	186	192	198	204	210	216
67	121	127	134	140	146	153	159	166	172	178	185	191	198	204	211	217	223
68	125	131	138	144	151	158	164	171	177	184	190	197	203	210	216	223	230
69	128	135	142	149	155	162	169	176	182	189	196	203	209	216	223	230	236
70	132	139	146	153	160	167	174	181	188	195	202	209	216	222	229	236	243
71	136	143	150	157	165	172	179	186	193	200	208	215	222	229	236	243	250
72	140	147	154	162	169	177	184	191	199	206	213	221	228	235	242	250	258
73	144	151	159	166	174	182	189	197	204	212	219	227	235	242	250	257	265
74	148	155	163	171	179	186	194	202	210	218	225	233	241	249	256	264	272
75	152	160	168	176	184	192	200	208	216	224	232	240	248	256	264	272	279
76	156	164	172	180	189	197	205	213	221	230	238	246	254	263	271	279	287

Figure 5: Body Mass Index (BMI) refers to an average number calculated from height and weight that typically correlates with body fat. BMI doesn't take into account muscle mass or body shape. Doctors use BMI to determine the risk for disease. Someone with a BMI below 19 is usually underweight. A BMI above 35 indicates "morbid" obesity. Obesity becomes morbid when it raises the risk of serious diseases (also known as co-morbidities).

CHAPTER 11
THE SUPER-SIZED METABOLIC SYNDROME

Our SAD, heavy in processed foods, soft drinks and fatty animal protein puts people at a much higher risk of developing metabolic syndrome, a dangerous cluster of disorders that occur at the same time and accelerate the progression of vascular disease. For the diagnosis of metabolic syndrome, a patient must have at least three related health conditions: significant belly fat, high blood pressure, insulin resistance, low HDL ("good") cholesterol levels, or elevated triglycerides. Metabolic syndrome may be referred to as Syndrome X, also known as pre-diabetes or insulin resistance syndrome. Doctors often do not recognize the cluster of related disorders if the patient's blood sugar and cholesterol levels are just a little high, or still within normal limits. It's the cluster of at least three of the "pre" conditions that increases the risk of vascular disease and diabetes.

Metabolic syndrome is primarily a nutritional disease caused by visceral fat, the omentum of belly fat packed deeply between organs. As we discussed in the previous chapter, the accumulation of excess weight, especially around the abdomen, generates inflammatory substances that increase the risk of insulin resistance, diabetes and vascular disease, among other illnesses. One of the largest research studies on metabolic syndrome found that our SAD of refined grains, processed lunch meat, fried food, red meat, eggs and soda, and less fish, fruit, vegetables and whole grains increased the risk of developing the triad of disorders characteristic of the syndrome.[67] This is another red flag that eating the wrong types of foods can cause, and even accelerate, the rate of disease. Diet was the singular most critical factor in the study, even when the researchers adjusted for the variables of smoking, caloric intake and physical activity.[68]

Pre-diabetes and Insulin Resistance

Insulin resistance is one of the driving forces of metabolic syndrome. If your average glucose fasting level rises above 100 milligrams per deciliter, you may have insulin resistance or "pre-diabetes." About 54 million adult Americans have pre-diabetes, according to the American Diabetes Association (ADA). Without

Diagnosing Metabolic Syndrome

The presence of 3 or more of these risk factors suggests metabolic syndrome

- Blood pressure 130/85 mm hg/higher
- Triglyceride 150 mg/dl/higher
- Fasting blood sugar 100 mg/dl/higher
- HDL less than 40 mg/dl (men); 50 mg/dl (women)
- Waistline 40 inches or more (men); 35 inches or more (women)

comprehensive lifestyle changes, pre-diabetes may become full-blown Type 2 diabetes in only 10 years.[69] Almost all individuals with Type 2 diabetes are insulin resistant.

Insulin is a hormone with multiple roles in our bodies, including transporting digested sugars (glucose) from the blood into cells for fuel, and fostering the storage of dietary fat into fat cells. Our brains are dependent on glucose to function properly. When we drink a soda that sharply raises blood glucose, our pancreas releases a surge of insulin to quickly restore the glucose to normal levels. When this happens, we feel a rush of energy followed by an equally large dip in energy and "brain fog" about an hour later.

With insulin resistance, cells don't respond normally to insulin, they've become resistant. Our pancreas reacts by churning out more and more insulin to help glucose get into our cells for energy. Too much glucose and insulin build up in our blood, creating the symptoms of diabetes—thirst, frequent urination, fatigue and hunger—and setting the stage for premature aging and disease. Excess insulin also increases the level of LDL cholesterol and triglycerides, as well as blood pressure and weight gain, raising the risk of stroke, heart attack and diabetes. As former president of the ADA, Francine Kaufman, M.D. noted in *Diabesity*, "The link between fat cells and inflammation helps explain the connection between obesity and [vascular] disease."[70] I first learned about metabolic syndrome several years ago when one of the hospital nurses in the ICU shared her symptoms with me.

Nancy was in her late 40s, a single mother who worked six days out of seven. Because we sometimes worked together in the ICU, she felt comfortable sharing her alarm about her increasing weight and decreasing energy level. At 195 pounds, with total cholesterol at 250, fasting glucose at 130, and blood pressure at 130/80, Nancy was on the fast track to a stroke or heart attack. She had metabolic syndrome.

Women with metabolic syndrome are at a much greater risk for premature vascular disease than men.

Making the rounds at the hospital to care for her many patients left Nancy feeling exhausted every day. Like most people with metabolic syndrome, she had the characteristic apple shape and carried around extra weight in her mid-section. She told me that her legs and back ached all the time, and if one of her ICU patients would "code," she would run into their room feeling a heart rate and breathlessness that seemed out of proportion to her level of exertion.

Nancy's doctor had prescribed a statin for her high cholesterol and blood pressure, and chided her for her obesity. She had refused to seek medical care ever since. When we met, first of all, I told her how impressed I was with her stamina in working full time in a demanding profession while raising three children on her own. Not very many people could handle the kind of stress she was dealt on a daily basis, and that is a fact. Then we got down to business. I asked her to describe a typical day in her life.

Nancy barely got by. I discovered that to compensate for her muscle aches and persistent fatigue, she would drink at least two 20-ounce bottles of *Coke*, take diet pills and over-the-counter pain relievers. She would also fast until dinnertime when she would typically order take-out and eat a large, kid-friendly American-Italian dinner like pizza, pasta or lasagna with her kids. Although she felt like her dinners were fine, given her daytime fasting and the demands of her job and home life, she was dead wrong.

With the combination of a slow metabolic rate from starving herself all day and the silent, diet-related inflammation festering in her body, it's no wonder that Nancy was feeling lousy. Rapidly digested refined

When Girth Matters	
Normal	**Risky**
Waist less than or equal to 40 inches (men) or 35 inches (women)	Waist greater than 40 inches (men) or 35 inches (women)

Figure 6: A wider girth increases the risk for heart attack, stroke, heart failure, diabetes and many common cancers.

carbohydrates like pasta or pizza don't provided enough nutrients or satiate our appetites like starchy whole foods. This means we end up eating larger portions to feel full, or return to the refrigerator later to snack. Simple carbohydrates also raise our blood glucose and insulin more than any other nutrient, a liability for someone on the cusp of developing Type 2 diabetes. High insulin levels promote fat storage and increase hunger. Belly fat also interferes with the effectiveness of insulin. What we choose to eat, weight we gain and the resulting metabolism reinforce each other.

Natural complex carbohydrates are healthier food choices. They provide vitamins, minerals, energy, and best of all, "resistant starch." Unprocessed foods are rich in resistant starch. As foods become more processed, like refined pasta or white bread, the amount of resistant starch decreases. Corn, peas, root vegetables such as yams, and fibrous fruits such as apples, pears and plantains turn off our appetites and turn up our metabolism. Legumes, brown rice and whole grains are other foods with resistant starch that increases our bodies' ability to burn fat. The nerves lining our digestive tract monitor the nutrient-density and calories of the food we eat. These nerves send the information to the hypothalamus in the brain which controls appetite and satiety. Tiny receptors sitting on top of cells in the stomach detect the volume of food eaten, not the weight. Nutrient-dense fiber from starch fills our gut and signals the brain that all is well, we can stop eating and start burning energy and fat.

The goal of the Non-Diet program is to reverse or eliminate the risk of vascular disease by healing and rebuilding metabolism through proper food selection, exercise and proven mind-body techniques. For anyone who would like to lose weight or reverse disease, spending time planning your weekly meals is a must. I told Nancy to start walking 30 minutes, five days a week and to begin eating small meals of starchy, fat-burning complex carbohydrates *consistently* every three to four hours. Consistency is one of the keys in rebuilding metabolism. When our bodies go without food for over four hours, our genetic response to starvation kicks in and metabolism slows down to conserve energy, making weight loss harder. The feast and famine way of eating works against powerful evolutionary forces.

Whether you're trying to lose weight or increase your energy level, breakfast is the most important meal of the day. Breakfast boosts your metabolism. If you consume only a small breakfast, such as a grapefruit or piece of wheat toast, then you'll need a mid-morning snack to keep your metabolism going strong. You should also stop eating three or four hours prior to bedtime. This raises your leptin levels, and actually burns fat while you sleep.

I also recommended to Nancy that she aggressively lower the percentage of fat in her diet to only 20 percent as long as she needed to lose weight, and then only 25 percent. For patients with metabolic syndrome at high risk for vascular disease, less than 5 percent of daily calories should come from saturated fat, and only 20-25 percent from total fat, provided that most of it is from unsaturated fat. Baked goods, pizza, beef, butter, whole milk and peanut butter are some of the fattiest foods. Consuming 100 calories of saturated fat converts to 97 calories of body fat. The fat you eat really is the fat you wear.

Finally, I asked Nancy to visualize what she would like to look or feel like on a daily basis. Write down your vision in a journal or draw a picture and put it where you can look at it every morning as a reminder, your brain will do the rest. Studies have shown that visualization and writing down your vision increases your ability to make it happen by programming your subconscious. Visualization is the language of the subconscious. Setting a timeline was also important. What did Nancy want to look like in three months, six months, etc.? Finally, I told her to set targets for her cholesterol, glucose and blood pressure levels too.

Several months went by without seeing Nancy, but she finally showed up in my office on a Friday afternoon in spring. Her weight was the first thing I noticed. She had lost over 65 pounds. "I feel 20 years younger," she said. She looked 20 years younger. Her hair seemed shinier and her skin definitely looked healthier. Best of all, her brown eyes had a new glint of life. Her lab results revealed that all of her numbers were back to normal, no more metabolic syndrome. She said that she no longer drank diet sodas or took medications, including pain relievers, and regularly walked during her lunch hour. Nancy was now healthier than the average person her age. But it was a gradual process that required consistent and comprehensive lifestyle changes, persistence, and the commitment that came from knowing that the changes would transform, and possibly even save her life.

Most people with a BMI over 35 have some degree of insulin resistance and metabolic syndrome. Doctors know that identifying metabolic syndrome in patients is far more effective than looking at BMI alone, as a way of predicting stroke and heart attack. If you're obese, you can cut your risk of metabolic syndrome and accelerated vascular disease by 80 percent if you lose only five percent of your body weight and exercise 30 minutes a day. Choosing nature's fat burners—complex carbohydrates with resistant starch—will help you lose weight faster. Many patients with metabolic syndrome think taking two or three drugs and insulin shots will shelter them from complications. But making comprehensive changes such as applying the rules and guidelines of the Non-Diet, daily exercise and practicing mind-body techniques, such as visualization, are the best strategies to eliminate the syndrome and reverse its dangerous effects.

Chapter 12

Diabetes: Not Your Grandmother's Disease

Up until 1997, the American Diabetes Association characterized Type 2 diabetes as a disease of the elderly. But the illness has increased multifold in obese young and middle-aged adults, teens and children, leading the association to revoke the term "adult-onset diabetes." The escalation of diabetes appears to be related to the increase in obesity rates. In 1958, less than 2 million Americans had diabetes. Today, about 10 percent, or 21 million, Americans have diabetes. An estimated one-third of Americans with Type 2 diabetes don't even know they have it. A combination of genetic and lifestyle factors trigger the disease. Immigrants from Latin America, Africa, South Asia and the Caribbean face a high risk of developing the disease when they move to North America. Minority populations, primarily African-Americans and Mexican-Americans, suffer the most from diabetes.[71]

Francine Kaufman, M.D., a pediatric endocrinologist and the former president of the American Diabetes Association, blamed the diabetes epidemic on "an economic structure that makes it cheaper to eat fries than fruit," and a food industry and mass media that lure children to eat the wrong foods and too much of them.[72] *The New York Times* health editor, Jane E. Brody, noted that a 15-year-long study published in *The Lancet* supports Dr. Kaufman's view. "A team headed by Dr. Mark A. Pereira of the University of Minnesota analyzed the eating habits of 3,031 young adults and found that weight gain and the development of pre-diabetes were directly related to unhealthful fast food."[73] Americans are paying the price for the glut of supersized food portions and sedentary lifestyles.

A Nutritional Disease

Diabetes affects the way our bodies use digested food for energy. As we discussed in the previous chapter, our bodies break down food into glucose, the form of sugar in the blood. Glucose is the main source of fuel for the body, especially the brain. People with diabetes have the incapacity to regulate blood glucose with the hormone insulin. Our pancreas secretes insulin to transport glucose into our cells, where it can be used for energy or stored in the form of glycogen in our liver or muscles. In uncontrolled diabetes, glucose and fats remain in the bloodstream and, over time, damage nerves, vital organs, and blood vessels, especially the sensitive endothelial cells that line the walls of arteries.

Obesity and diabetes go hand-in-hand. Visceral fat, as we learned in the chapter on obesity, generates bioactive substances that promote insulin resistance and inflammation, affecting every cell in the body. Chronic inflammation can cause even more damage to the artery's endothelium than plaque.

When our pancreas cannot produce insulin, triglyceride levels rise and may cause the arteries to constrict. This decreases blood flow to the heart, brain, and kidneys, and increases the risk of pulmonary embolism, heart attack and stroke. Excess glucose also contributes to neuropathy and peripheral vascular disease that can result in blindness and lower-extremity amputations.

Type 1 and Type 2 diabetes mellitus also causes a condition called diabetic nephropathy, which is the leading cause of kidney disease in the United States. Many doctors recommend a low-protein food program like the Non-Diet for patients whose kidneys are deteriorating. A diabetic's need for kidney dialysis is common. Vascular disease is the leading cause of diabetes-related deaths. Rates of death are about two to four times higher for adults with diabetes than for those without the disease.

The Different Types of Diabetes

There are two main types of diabetes. Type 1 diabetes often appears during childhood or adolescence and involves the child of a parent, brother or sister with diabetes. In Type 1, the immune system destroys insulin-producing beta cells in the pancreas and makes patients dependent on frequent insulin injections to keep the body's blood sugar under control. The cause is unknown. When the disease isn't under control, diabetics can experience the increased need to urinate, hunger and thirst, weight loss, blurred vision, weakness and fatigue, irritability and frequent infections. Type 1 diabetics tend to be thin. When the pancreas produces no insulin, sugar cannot be used for energy and the body burns fat for its energy. A century ago insulin-diabetic children usually died young. Now they can live a normal life if they take insulin medication, exercise and follow a reasonable diet. Only about 5 to 10 percent of people with diabetes have Type 1.

Type 2 diabetes (non-insulin dependent) most often appears in people older than 40. Though doctors are diagnosing more and more young people with the life-long disorder. Type 2 diabetes accounts for 90 percent of all U.S. cases, and develops more often in overweight and sedentary people. The risk of Type 2 diabetes is 1.6 times as great for blacks as for whites of a similar age, and twice as great for Mexican-Americans and Native Americans.

High-Glycemic Foods
- Bagels
- Cake
- Candy bars
- Couscous
- Cranberry juice cocktail
- French fries
- Jelly beans
- Mashed potatoes
- Pancakes
- Refined breakfast cereals
- Strawberry jam
- Sugar-sweetened beverages
- White bread
- White pasta
- White rice

A Type 2 diabetic produces insulin, but the body has developed a resistance to it. Insulin resistance, as we learned in the chapter on metabolic syndrome, means that insulin cannot get inside cells to produce or store energy. Since the cells are not getting the insulin they need, the pancreas produces more and more insulin to compensate, resulting in abnormally high levels of insulin and sugar in the blood.

Diabetes has far-reaching effects on our bodies and can lead to serious complications. These complications include lower extremity amputation, kidney disease, cognitive decline and premature death from stroke, heart attack, kidney or heart failure. Diabetes is the sixth leading cause of preventable death. But patients who make even modest lifestyle changes can prevent these dire complications. While medications may be necessary for some, ramping up the exercise routine and following the Non-Diet way of eating can effectively treat, and even reverse the disease for others.

A Nutritional Cure

You can reduce your odds of developing Type 2 diabetes by carrying a normal weight and avoiding high-glycemic foods such as refined carbohydrates and sugar, and by eating a complex carbohydrate diet that includes whole grains. These foods stimulate the pancreas to secrete insulin.

Foods contain three major types of nutrients: carbohydrates, proteins and fats. Complex carbohydrates, such as fruits, vegetables, legumes and grains, come from plants. The resistant fiber in complex carbohydrates lowers cholesterol, slows glucose absorption and controls the rate of digestion.

If you follow the recommendations of the USDA food pyramid, six to eleven servings of refined (white) bread, rice and pasta, you would be eating a diet rich in simple carbohydrates but extremely low in nutrients. This is the same SAD that fueled our epidemic of obesity, metabolic syndrome, diabetes and vascular disease in the first place. A 2007 study from Harvard University found that people who ate whole-grain foods on a regular basis were one-third less likely to develop metabolic syndrome, diabetes or vascular disease, compared to those who rarely ate whole-grain foods.[74]

People who are overweight have a much higher risk of diabetes because, as we learned, fat interferes with the body's ability to use insulin. Advocates of the Atkins and other high-protein diets claim that their approach to losing weight is especially good for people with diabetes. The Nutrition Council of the AHA countered, "A very-high-protein diet is especially risky for patients with diabetes, because it can speed the progression, even for short lengths of time, of diabetic renal disease."[75]

High-protein diets are restrictive of carbohydrate choices and liberal with protein choices, even though meat is associated with artery-clogging saturated fat and cholesterol. These diets also do not offer a variety of nutrient-dense foods, especially the starchy complex carbohydrates needed to slow digestion and adequately meet nutritional needs.

Doctors consider a fasting blood sugar of 110 to 125 as borderline or pre-diabetes, above 125 may be full-blown diabetes. Type 2 diabetics typically have high blood pressure, and HDL cholesterol of less than 35 or triglyceride level of greater than 250. Be sure to ask your doctor to run a lipid profile and repeat your fasting glucose test before making a final diagnosis. And because blood sugar levels vary throughout the day, ask for the HbA1c blood test.

The HbA1c blood test measures the level of sugar attached to your red blood cells over a three to four month period, the average lifetime of a red blood cell. If you don't have tight control over your diabetes, your red blood cells will accumulate sugar. See Figure 6 to gauge your level of sugar control in your blood with two different tests.

Daily Glucose	Quarterly HbA1c	Goal
90 mg/dl	5	Excellent
150 mg/dl	7	Good
210 mg/dl	9	Fair
240 mg/dl	10	Poor
360 mg/dl	14	Failing

Figure 7: Daily/Quarterly Glucose Checks

Diabetes Control

The most important treatment for diabetes is strict control of blood glucose levels via nutrition, exercise and regular blood glucose testing. If lifestyle changes are insufficient, you may require daily insulin injections. Type 2 diabetes is largely a nutritional and lifestyle-driven disease.

A dietitian or nutritionist can provide invaluable help as you develop a personalized eating plan based on the secrets of the Non-Diet and the advice of your doctor. After all, you're not making temporary adjustments, this is a lifelong commitment. Learning how to prevent or treat hypoglycemia, if it occurs, is a critical health issue to discuss with your doctor. People newly diagnosed with Type 2 diabetics are usually asked to keep a food diary to track their calories, carbohydrates and fats. I also recommend that patients write their feelings down as they adjust to the "new normal." Using the mind body techniques recommended in the previous chapter is valuable too, especially when making comprehensive changes to your life. The good news is that Type 2 diabetes is reversible. The Non-Diet was designed to help patients with the disease.

Several studies support that insulin resistance and diabetes have a strong relationship with excessive weight. For instance, the NIH-sponsored Diabetes Prevention Program studied over 3,000 American adults at high risk for developing Type 2 diabetes due to obesity and elevated blood sugar levels. The researchers found that only modest lifestyle changes, including five to seven pounds of weight loss and 30 minutes of exercise five times weekly, reduced the risk of diabetes by 58 percent.[76] The key take-away is that even modest weight loss and exercise can delay, if not prevent or reverse, diabetes in many people who take on the Herculean task of changing their life.

Chapter 13
Under Pressure with Hypertension

Over 73 million Americans have hypertension (high blood pressure), a disease that is twice as common among people who are obese than among those who are not. The more you weigh, the greater the risk of developing hypertension and its complications: stroke, heart attack, heart failure and, most of all, chronic kidney disease. Chronic kidney disease is especially prevalent among African-Americans. Over four million Americans are estimated to have kidney disease caused by high blood pressure. According to the NIH, African-Americans are six times more likely than whites to develop kidney failure from hypertension.[77] Treating hypertension with medication alone is not enough, according to a recent study.

Following the Non-Diet way of eating, exercising and learning how to cope better with stress can help prevent or reverse high blood pressure. Only 30 to 60 minutes of exercise, 3-4 days a week can lower your blood pressure by 4 to 9 millimeters of mercury (mm Hg). By exercising and losing weight you may be able to avoid expensive medications and potential complications. Every 2.2 pounds of weight you lose results in a corresponding drop of roughly one mm systolic pressure, the top number in a blood pressure reading which measures the maximum arterial pressure when the heart muscle contracts. Every 2.2 pounds of weight you lose results in a corresponding drop of roughly 1 mm diastolic pressure, the bottom number which measures the minimum arterial pressure when the heart is at rest. Cutting back on salt can lower blood pressure too.[78]

Hypertension and Vascular Disease

Blood pressure medication has a minimal effect in reducing heart attacks because it does not remove the underlying problem, plaque formation. When you exert yourself chemical messengers like epinephrine travel in the nervous system to alert your heart and coronary arteries to respond to your needs. If the coronary arteries contract, blood pressure rises. If the arteries dilate to a larger diameter, blood pressure falls. The messengers that raise blood pressure also trigger the release of angiotensin II that inflames arteries and triggers the growth of plaque.

Over time, hypertension actually causes vascular disease which stiffens the arteries, weakening their ability to respond to the increased demand of your activities. If you have severe vascular disease you may feel chest pain, fatigue or shortness of breath when attempting to exert yourself. When arteries become stiffer they can bulge and rupture or become inflamed and dysfunctional, increasing the risk of heart attack, aneurysm, stroke and heart or kidney damage. Taking medication without changing your lifestyle can kill you.

The Silent Killer

Unlike other medical conditions, hypertension progresses silently, increasing year to year with or without recognizable signs or symptoms. If symptoms do appear they can include chest pain, swelling of the ankles and feet, headaches, fatigue, ringing in the ears, visual changes, facial flushing or the loss of concentration and memory.

Several factors affect your blood pressure: the volume of fluid in your blood, the diameter of your blood vessels, and the force of your heart contractions. Blood pressure is the force needed to move blood throughout your vascular system. Doctors use two numbers to measure blood pressure: the systolic pressure (as the heart beats) over the diastolic pressure (as the heart relaxes between beats). Blood pressure is written as systolic pressure/diastolic pressure, for example 120/80 mm Hg (millimeters of mercury). Normal blood pressure is less than 120 mm Hg systolic and less than 80 mm Hg diastolic. From a clinical perspective, systolic and diastolic pressures are of equal importance.

The risk for strokes and heart attacks actually starts at 115/75. The higher the blood pressure, the greater the risks are for complications. In most people with high blood pressure, both systolic and diastolic pressures are high. The exception is older people who typically have high systolic pressure (140 mm Hg or more) with normal or low diastolic pressure (less than 90 mm Hg).

According to the AHA, only 5-10 percent of people with high blood pressure have a known condition causing the illness such as a kidney abnormality, congenital defect of the aorta or narrowing of certain arteries. Hypertension is deadly if not treated and occurs more often in African-Americans.

When I was a resident in neurosurgery at Georgetown University and Washington General, I would often have to operate on African-

Americans with blood pressure related brain bleeds. High blood pressure often occurs earlier in life. It is more severe and has more complications in African-Americans. And yet, blacks are less likely to seek treatment until their blood pressure has been high for so long that vital organs have already started to suffer damage. Denial is often a component in seeking treatment, but so are lack of access to medical care, misdiagnosis, lack of awareness about preventive self-care and dismissive doctors.[79]

Women face even greater obstacles and may have no feeling of empowerment when it comes to preventative health care, and for good reason. Several studies have shown that physicians don't listen as well, preventative medications aren't prescribed as often, diagnostic tests aren't as accurate and women's symptoms are harder to recognize.[80]

What Causes High Blood Pressure?

According to the AHA, in about 95 percent of high blood pressure cases, the cause is unknown and the patient may feel no symptoms. About 5-10 percent of people with high blood pressure have a condition causing the illness:
• Kidney abnormality
• A structural abnormality of the aorta, the large blood vessel leaving the heart, existing since birth
• Narrowing of certain arteries

Blood Pressure and Diet

Blood pressure increases with age, especially in Western countries such as the U.S. where a high-sodium, fatty diet, chronic stress and inactivity are prevalent. Rates of hypertension are low in developing countries such as China, possibly because the traditional Chinese plant-based diet is lower in sodium.[81]

Nine out of 10 Americans will develop high blood pressure, and many may not even be aware that they have the condition. One of my patients, 48-year-old Lisa, thought she was losing her mind before we discovered that her symptoms were due to out-of-control blood pressure. Uncontrolled high blood pressure contributes to mild cognitive impairment which causes learning, memory and thinking difficulties.

The only test for hypertension is a blood pressure measurement. You should take several blood pressure readings with an at-home monitor before making a final conclusion. Sit down for a few minutes before taking the test. Blood pressure rises with weight, activity and time of day. You can purchase an inexpensive blood pressure monitor at a drug store and it may save your life.

Only one-third of Americans who have hypertension have it under control. Over time, high blood pressure can actually cause severe vascular disease. The first complication may be a heart attack, stroke or aneurysm. Unfortunately, I see too many fatal brain aneurysms from untreated hypertension.

Often, dietary and other lifestyle changes are sufficient to keep blood pressure controlled. If not, it may be necessary to add blood pressure medications such as diuretics, ACE inhibitors, beta blockers or calcium channel blockers. In choosing an anti-hypertensive drug, doctors consider such factors as the person's age, sex and race. They also consider the severity of high blood pressure, the presence of other conditions such as diabetes or high blood cholesterol levels, potential side effects, varying from drug to drug, and the costs of the drugs and of tests needed to check for certain side effects. Physicians consider patients with a blood pressure of 120/80 to 139/89 as pre-hypertensive and at high risk for hypertension.

According to the prestigious Mayo Clinic, a blood pressure of 115/75 mm Hg should be the gold standard. Even someone in their 30s or younger who has hypertension has *five times* the risk of heart attack than someone with normal blood pressure. Losing as few as 10 pounds can lower blood pressure. Primary hypertension, hypertension that isn't secondary to an adrenal tumor or other medical condition, cannot be cured, it can be controlled to prevent complications. See the chart below to check your blood pressure.

Category	Systolic (mmg)	Diastolic (mmg)
Normal blood pressure	115	75
High-normal blood pressure	Below 130	Below 85
Stage 1 hypertension	140-159	90-99
Stage 2 hypertension	160-179	100-109
Stage 3 hypertension	180 or higher	110 or higher

Figure 8: Measuring Adult Blood Pressure (Source: Merck)

Taking Its Toll

According to the AHA, one in three American adults has high blood pressure. In 2004 the death rates per 100,000 people from high blood pressure were 15.7 for white males, 51.0 for black males, 14.5 for white females and 40.9 for black females.[82] When pressure in the arteries is above 140/90 mm Hg, the heart enlarges and the heart's walls thicken because the heart has to work harder to pump blood. Consequently, the heart's chambers do not expand normally and are harder to fill with blood, further increasing the heart's workload. These changes in the heart may result in abnormal heart rhythms or even heart failure.

Making simple changes such as exercising, reducing the amount of alcohol you drink and throwing out the salt shaker may make drug therapy unnecessary. Daily alcohol intake should be reduced to no more than two drinks, and sodium intake should be reduced to less than two grams. People with primary hypertension don't have to restrict their physical activity as long as their blood pressure is under control.

Diets high in sodium, fat and carbohydrates are known to exacerbate blood pressure and the strain on blood vessels, arteries, heart, brain and kidneys. If we eat the wrong kinds of foods over many years, certain chemicals are activated that contribute to vascular disease. Research clearly shows that exercise and losing weight reduces blood glucose and blood pressure, HDL also goes up and inflammation levels drop. Weight reduction has a tremendous impact on high blood pressure. Eating fiber-rich fruits and vegetables also lowers blood pressure.

The level of stress in your life influences your blood pressure too. Strong emotional states such as anger and hostility can raise blood pressure and even wreak havoc with the heart's sensitive electrical system. Workers who are under constant stress may start to show it through their blood pressure readings. In a study that followed more than 6,719 white-collar

> **Dietary Approaches to Stop Hypertension (DASH):**
> - Emphasize fruits and vegetables. Daily goal is 5 servings of fruit and 4 servings of vegetables daily
> - Choose non or low-fat dairy products
> - Choose whole-grain breads and cereals
> - Eat walnuts and almonds
> - Reduce intake of red meats, sweets and sodas

Risk of Complications
Controlling elevated blood pressure can cut strokes by 35 to 40 percent and heart attacks by 20 to 25 percent (Source: AHA)

workers for 7.5 years, Canadian researchers found that those with high job demands and low levels of social support tended to have higher blood pressure than other workers.[83] Better social networks can cast a net under workers suffering from stress.

The risks associated with untreated high blood pressure are daunting. These risks include heart failure, heart attack, sudden cardiac death, kidney failure and stroke. In fact, high blood pressure is the most important risk factor that a person can control to prevent premature heart failure, stroke or heart attack. The bottom line is that it's up to you. See your doctor yearly to check your blood pressure. Exercise, eat lots of fiber-rich foods and learn how to better manage day-to-day stress with mind body techniques such as breathing exercises and visualization. Without lifestyle changes, especially weight loss, few people living with hypertension can live a normal lifespan. But today, thanks to our knowledge about modifiable behaviors and medications, many people can change the course of the disease.

CHAPTER 14
SMOKING: LIGHTING UP INFLAMMATION

In the early morning hours of October 28, 2007, a deadly blaze quietly consumed the lives of seven college students who were sleeping soundly in their beds at a beach house in North Carolina. State and federal investigators concluded that careless smoking was the most likely cause. Most people think of lung cancer when they think about smoking and death. But smoking is responsible for 40 percent of all house fires. A quick Google search on "house fires smoking children," sadly reveals how often the main victims of house fires are the children of smokers.

Another surprising statistic is that almost half of all vascular deaths, heart attack, stroke, arrhythmias, pulmonary embolism or heart failure, are related to tobacco use. Cigarettes, smokeless tobacco and pipe tobacco are loaded with numerous toxic chemicals. A lighted cigarette gives off several *thousand* chemical compounds in the form of gases and particles, including 45 known carcinogens such as nicotine, also used as an insecticide to kill bugs, carbon monoxide, the same gas in car exhaust, tar, the same stuff used to pave highways, and hydrogen cyanide, also used as gas chamber poison. Nicotine and carbon monoxide are the chief toxins in a burning cigarette.

Every day about 15 billion cigarettes are smoked across the globe, more than two for every human-being alive. Over 21 million Americans smoke, according to the CDC. The risk of vascular disease for a tobacco user is much greater than the risk of lung cancer, and greatly increases with the number of cigarettes smoked daily. If you begin smoking as a teenager, as the majority of smokers do, you lose 20 seconds of your life with each cigarette you smoke. People who smoke a pack a day die, on average, seven years earlier than people who have never smoked.

Vascular disease is far more extensive in smokers than non-smokers. Smoking injures the smooth inner muscle of arteries, causing the build-up of plaque and endothelial dysfunction, which can lead to coronary spasms, ischemia (lack of blood flow) and arrhythmia. Nicotine can trigger the development of blood clots which may result in stroke, pulmonary embolism or heart attack. Smokers are five times more likely to die from sudden cardiac death than non-smokers. About five years after quitting, ex-smokers have a 50 percent reduction in the risk for heart attack, stroke and a fatal blood clot in the lungs.

When I was resident at Georgetown University hospital, a young college student complaining of left calf pain and swelling came to the emergency room. She had a beautiful smile, stark blue eyes and dark black hair which reminded me of Carolyn, my first wife. On exam, her left calf was swollen and tender. She jumped when I touched it. I also listened to her lungs and discovered that she was wheezing. She said she didn't have asthma or a cold. Her heart rhythm was steady and normal.

Although rare, I suspected deep vein thrombosis (DVT) and a blood clot that had traveled into the lung, becoming a pulmonary embolism (PE). A large PE can plug the great vessels of the lung, halting blood flow out of the heart's right ventricle and causing a rapid death. PE's are hard to detect. Wheezing or coughing, chest pain and lower leg pain are the most common symptoms that may precede a large, catastrophic blood clot. Despite discouragement from my supervisor, I erred on the side of caution and ordered a pulmonary angiogram because she smoked and was taking birth control pills, which had only been on the market for a few years at that time. My suspicions were correct. The X-ray revealed several clots in her lungs and I admitted her to the hospital where she was put on a blood thinner. Even though today's birth control pills are safer, women who smoke and take the pill are almost 10 times as likely to die from blood clots as non-smokers.

Up in Smoke

Nicotine raises blood pressure about 15 points and increases heart rate by about 20 beats per minute, increasing the workload on the heart. Blood pressure, pulse rate and breathing patterns start returning to normal soon after quitting. Carbon monoxide levels in the blood drop, oxygen levels increase and nerve endings begin to re-grow, decreasing the risk of serious nerve diseases that mainly affect the eyes, brain and limbs.

Besides bad breath and smelly clothes, smoking also causes premature aging. The chemicals in tobacco smoke narrow the blood vessels in the outermost layers of the skin, impairing blood flow. The depletion of oxygen and important nutrients, such as vitamin A, also damages collagen and elastin. These fibers that give skin its strength and elasticity, especially in women's breasts. As a result, skin begins to sag and wrinkle prematurely. Heavy smokers typically look 10 years older than they really are.

Smokers may think that they're relieving stress by smoking a cigarette. But they are actually stimulating the part of the nervous system involved in the body's stress response, the autonomic nervous system (ANS). Lighting up a cigarette is like lighting up the whole body with stress. Repeated exposure to the stress response causes chemical changes in the body that lead to chronic inflammation, the chief cause of smoking-related disease and illness.

Second-Hand Smoke Kills

Nearly half of all chronic smokers die an average of 20 to 25 years before their time. One of the most devastating facts is that second-hand smoke often kills innocent bystanders: the smoker's wife or husband, daughter or son. I'll never forget what my 43-year-old patient, Angie, shouted as I stepped into the examining room two years ago "Back pain is ruining my life! It's ruining my life, Dr. Kachmann!" I also remember being hit by the odor of smoke and noticed, in the back of my mind, that Rick, Angie's husband, had the haggard, worn look of a heavy smoker. He had sat in the chair beside the examining table, opening and closing his palms in a gesture of nervous impatience. Angie joked that she had been married to Rick for 15 years, 15 of which she had begged him to quit smoking. She was a dental assistant. They had one child, a boy in fourth grade.

I liked Angie and worried that her symptoms indicated something more serious than the usual back problems because of the severity of her pain. Low back pain can be quite debilitating and painful. But I thought Angie's complaints were unusually dramatic. After performing a routine neurological exam, I ordered a bone scan, chest X-ray and CT of the lungs and abdomen, tests that I rarely order to investigate low back pain.

Much to my horror and great sadness, the X-rays revealed diffuse, end-stage lung cancer that had spread to the liver and the sacrum, her lower spine. Angie died within six months and, quite frankly, I believe her husband's smoking was responsible. Secondhand smoke can kill.

The Mind of Addiction

Many substances and activities, from food to sex, exert control over human behavior by motivating us to indulge in them. But addictive drugs, such as alcohol, nicotine, cocaine and heroin, can affect the structure and function of the brain and hence our motivations in long-lasting ways. They can actually alter and usurp the "circuits" in the brain that are involved in the control of emotions and motivation, impairing an addicted person's will. Addiction really is the result of brain changes that, over time, get translated into behavior changes.

All drugs of abuse, from alcohol to nicotine to heroin, cause a series of temporary changes in the brain that produce the "high." One of these changes is the rise in available levels of certain neurotransmitters associated with feelings of pleasure. Key among these is dopamine, a naturally occurring neurotransmitter that some scientists now think is implicated in most of the basic human experiences of pleasure. The pleasure of a kiss, a bowl of favorite ice cream or a compliment may all be related to a rise in dopamine levels in the normal person's brain. When a person takes a hit of crack cocaine or a drag on a cigarette, the drug causes a spike in dopamine levels in the brain and a rush of euphoria, or pleasure. While it's not the only chemical involved in drug abuse, experts have come to believe that dopamine is the crucial one.

Nicotine addiction also changes the way nerve cells in the brain communicate in such a way that smokers develop compulsive, out-of-control-type behavior. This happens despite knowing that all kinds of terrible things can happen as a result of their habit, and despite experiencing many of those things. Most Americans have been affected in some way by addiction to drugs of abuse like nicotine, such as witnessing a loved one die of a smoking-related illness. Yet addiction to nicotine is a phenomenon that has been clouded by myth, misunderstanding and moral judgments. The very nature of the problem, what addiction is, has long been debated. Most people probably continue to think of addiction, particularly to illicit drugs, as primarily a moral or character problem, something caused by degeneracy or lack of willpower. However, scientific research into addiction has led experts to conclude that addiction is actually a disease, a chronic illness like diabetes or hypertension. The so-called disease model doesn't mean that addicts cannot stop using nicotine, only that doing so is difficult and often requires medical treatment and major lifestyle changes.

Scientists and medical experts now consider the *disease* of nicotine addiction to be chronic and relapsing. From a clinical point of view addiction is more like hypertension, which requires long-term treatment with medication and lifestyle changes, unlike a broken bone which is set, healed and forgotten. People recovering from addiction are advised to avoid people and places associated with their drug-using behavior.

Nicotine addiction is a disease that causes physiological changes in the brain which then drive certain behaviors, such as smoking in secret or smoking compulsively. However, addicts can learn to change the behavior. Treatment of and recovery from addiction is possible. Steven Hyman, M.D., who directs the National Institute of Mental Health, compares the disease of addiction to heart disease, which may also necessitate major lifestyle changes. We shouldn't blame smokers for the disease. But we should treat them as having responsibility for their recovery.

Recovering from Nicotine Addiction

A year ago, I walked onto a New York subway platform and saw a poster of a smoker who had his larynx removed and speaks through an artificial voice box that said, "Smoking gave me throat cancer at age 39. Now I breathe through a hole in my throat and need this machine to speak." According to *The New York Times*, the poster prompted a threefold increase in calls to the New York City Department of Health and Mental Hygiene from people interested in smoking cessation programs.

If you're using tobacco to lose weight, think again, smoking is the single worst thing you can do for your health and the most preventable cause of death. If you've tried to quit before and failed, it's time to summon your resolve and try again. Nicotine withdrawal symptoms subside within five days. The chemicals have left the body within 21 days, especially if you drink a lot of water.

Within our personal chemistry we carry a medicine that reduces stress and prevents depression, even more effectively than any drug. Keep yourself busy and reward yourself with massage or yoga. Munching on healthy snacks such as celery helps. Exercise, music, humor and visualization also help the brain overcome addiction. Imagine yourself without a cigarette in your hand and visualize all the aspects of your life that will change without cigarettes: no more alienation from restaurants and other public places that ban smoking; fresh breath; more energy and better skin; smoke-free clothes; more money in your pocket; and most of all, a better quality of life and a longer life expectancy.

CHAPTER 15

AEROBIC FITNESS AND LONGEVITY

Your aerobic fitness is a key indicator of vascular health and longevity. Your lifespan increases when you burn more than 2,000 calories a week on exercise. Sitting in a chair, your heart is beating at only 42 percent of its maximum rate. At that level, there's no benefit. Walking burns about 300 calories per hour. If you walk six hours per week, you'll burn all the calories you need to get the vascular benefits to reduce your overall threat of dying before your time. Higher intensity exercises, like biking, burn about twice the amount of calories per hour. But simply jogging or biking one-and-a-half hours per week will not burn as many calories as six days of 30-60 minutes of walking. Although you get the benefit of calorie burning from rowing, tennis or jogging much faster, walking is just as efficient.

Regular aerobic activity develops your aerobic fitness, your heart and lungs' capacity to process oxygen. A treadmill test with a face mask and EKG, administered by a cardiologist, is the gold standard for measuring your overall aerobic fitness. The test measures breathing and heart rates in about 10 to 15 minutes. The results are expressed in metabolic equivalents of task, or METs, a numerical rating of the body's ability to produce energy needed to perform certain activities. The greater the activity, the greater the number of METs needed.

Your doctor may refer to a treadmill test like this as an Exercise Tolerance Test or Exercise Stress Test. At three-minute intervals, the speed and the incline of the treadmill increase. The test starts at 2.74km/hr at a gradient, or incline, of 10 percent. At minute three the speed increases to 4.02km/hr and the gradient increases to 12 percent. This is a maximal test, which means that you continue the test until you feel fatigued. In a clinical setting, other parameters such as shortness of breath, chest pain, high blood pressure or disturbing ECG reading may determine the end of the test. See Figure 7 for the standard aerobic fitness levels correlated with time, speed and gradient variables.

The Bruce Treadmill Test Protocol			
Level	Time (mins)	Speed (km/hr)	Grade (%)
1	0	2.74	10
2	3	4.02	12
3	6	5.47	14
4	9	6.76	16
5	12	8.05	18
6	15	8.85	20
7	18	9.65	22

Figure 9: Measuring Aerobic Fitness

The average man or woman has a range of eight to 12 METs capacity. Marathon runners have generally 15 to 20 METs. The elderly, patients with vascular disease, the obese or unfit may average five to eight METs. Increasing your maximal MET level is crucial for cardiac health and longevity. The higher the MET level, the lower the death rate from vascular disease or cancer. Walking briskly for 30 minutes is a good way to improve your MET level. A low MET level is the strongest predictor of mortality. The treadmill test costs about $500 and is not totally without risk. A doctor should be nearby. Most people who can briskly walk 30 minutes a day can attain a cardio-protective fitness level of nine to 10 METs or more.

Exercise is a must for patients who have suffered a heart attack, stroke, have been diagnosed with vascular disease or one of the cancers listed on pages 37 or page 145. A study of British men with coronary artery disease revealed that those who participated in moderate exercise, at least 40 minutes of walking per day, were 58 percent less likely to die from any cause over the five years of research.[84] Many studies have proven that lifestyle changes, including improved nutrition, no smoking and moderate exercise, can reduce vascular disease risk more effectively than most drugs.

Research from the Women's Health Study found that participants who burned at least 1,000 calories a week with physical activity were less likely to have a heart attack, bypass surgery or angioplasty. The risk of dying from heart disease grew with decreasing activity and increasing weight. Exercise lowers blood pressure, insulin and glucose levels, and helps prevent blood clots and stroke (the number one cause of disability in women and men).

Regular exercise will add years to your life, especially if you're already dealing with a chronic disease or recovering from cancer, heart attack or stroke. You gain about *two hours* of life expectancy for every hour of aerobic exercise. Another benefit is that depression is much less common in people who exercise. Aerobic exercise triggers the release of endorphins, our natural pain killers. Exercise will even make you smarter by increasing the number of brain cells in certain regions of the brain, notably the frontal lobes, our "executive center" for planning, decision-making and concentration. A prescription for regular aerobic exercise is a key part of the Non-Diet program for vitality and optimal health.

Chapter 16

The Mind-Body Connection to Health

Our ability to cope with stress has far-reaching biological impacts. Under stress, the body shuts down resources from the immune, digestive and endocrine systems and releases hormones from the nervous and circulatory systems that fuel the body to act. The stress response is fundamentally influenced by brain function and neurochemicals that also trigger inflammatory mechanisms known to influence the development of hypertension and vascular disease. In other words, stress is a toxin that can kill. Long-term stress can cause an "over-reaction" by the body's immune system, which causes inflammation in vascular tissues. Sometimes stress damages our bodies at a steady rate over many years, other times suddenly. We're more susceptible to illness when under stress, especially when we're bombarded all day long with situations that we *perceive* as stressful. Psychological stress has a tremendous effect on the heart, the center of our circulatory system.

The writer John Gregory Dunne had a sudden, fatal heart attack, just as he and his wife had returned home from visiting their deathly-ill daughter in the Intensive Care Unit. Joan Didion wrote about the year of grieving after her husband's death in *The Year of Magical Thinking*.[85] And who can forget Kenneth Lay, the founder of Enron who faced the possibility of life in prison for fraud and conspiracy, dying of a heart attack just before his sentencing?[86] Most sudden deaths occur because blood pressure rises and electrical impulses become rapid (ventricular tachycardia) or chaotic (ventricular fibrillation).

If you look at the chief risk factors for vascular disease, inflammation, LDL cholesterol, diabetes, and hypertension, stress doesn't seem as harmful in comparison. But the accumulative effect of stress is inflammation that damages blood vessels and vital organs. The physiology of stress and the "fight-or-flight" response has been studied more than any other neurochemical process.

When the brain perceives something as stressful, a quick swerve in the traffic ahead or a toddler teetering on the edge of the stairs, the adrenal glands produce cortisol to raise blood sugar and fuel the muscles to run, even if we don't go anywhere. The kidneys also produce aldosterone, a steroid hormone that raises blood pressure. Stress also triggers the brain's hypothalamus to release adrenaline, noradrenalin and related chemicals. These raise cholesterol, constrict blood vessels and increase heart rate, all of which may cause skipped heartbeats, tremors, chest pain and that anxious feeling of apprehension. Adrenaline is even known to make platelets stickier, increasing blood clotting.

The stress response often acts as a trigger for sudden death when conditions such as hypertension, obesity, vascular disease or cardiomyopathy are present. Life-threatening arrhythmias doubled in a group of implantable cardioverter defibrillators (ICDs) recipients in the month after the September 11 attacks.[87] ICDs, or fibrillation, are used in heart patients at risk for recurrent, sustained ventricular tachycardia to deliver electrical shocks, sense the cardiac rhythm and sometimes pace the heart.

The emotional part of our brain develops in vitro before the "executive center," the frontal cortex, which aids in planning and decision-making. The fact that we are emotional before we are rational is most obvious during sports events like the Super Bowl or World Cup. The pandemonium of rivaling teams can lead to anxiety, panic and even cardiac arrest in fans with no prior history of vascular disease. Eleven soccer fans died of cardiac arrest in China during the 2006 World Cup. Chinese officials tagged it the "World Cup Syndrome."

Heart Intelligence

Negative emotions throw our nervous system out of balance. Researchers at the Heart Math Institute for neuralcardiology experimented with heart rate variability, or heart rhythms, to gauge emotional states and stress. When subjects in the studies focused on feelings such as anger or sadness, their heart rhythms appeared jagged and chaotic. When they focused on love or appreciation, the heart converted to a slower and steadier rhythm. Emotion generates physiological changes in the heart.

The heart even has a mind of its own. Specialized neural circuits with clusters of nerve cells and neurotransmitters exist within the heart muscle. The heart even emits an energy field that can be measured more than 10 feet away from the body.[88] The neural, biochemical and electromagnetic messages that the heart generates and transmits to the brain have a profound influence on our physiological, mental and emotional health.

Many studies have examined the link between vascular disease and job strain, typically defined as work with high psychological demands but with little decision-making authority. Jobs such as an assembly-line worker, garment worker, waiter and cook have high demands and low control, and are known to have much higher rates of heart attack than white-collar managerial jobs.

It's well-known in Emergency Medicine that life-threatening heart arrhythmias, heart attacks and strokes occur more often at the beginning or end of the work week. Stress constricts blood vessels, which raises blood pressure and makes it harder for the heart to pump blood. Workers who are under constant stress may start to show it in their blood pressure readings.

Stress can even "break" your heart. "Broken heart syndrome" is a rare cardiac disorder that mimics a heart attack. Some people, especially women, may respond to sudden, overwhelming emotional stress such as the death of a loved one, car accident or even the intense emotional stress of a wedding or surprise party by releasing large amounts of adrenaline, cortisol and other potent chemicals into the blood stream. These chemicals can be temporarily toxic to the heart, effectively stunning the muscle and producing symptoms similar to a heart attack or heart failure: chest discomfort, sweating, shortness of breath and swelling.

Stress isn't the only emotion with the potential to do harm. Anger is the most toxic emotion for the heart, increasing the risk of a heart attack by 230 percent. Two people can be in the same room, facing the same situation but may perceive it differently. "We boil at different degrees," said philosopher Ralph Waldo Emerson. The risk of heart attack in people who are impatient or lose their temper is five to seven times higher than someone who has learned better coping strategies. If you're driven and tend to feel a great sense of urgency, be sure to increase your exercise, meditate or learn to appreciate music and art. Seek activities that quiet your mind. The goal is to get your head and heart in sync.

The combination of hostility plus depression appears to be as dangerous a risk factor for vascular disease as high blood pressure or even smoking. The Greek word meaning "constriction" is the root of "anger" and "angina." When a person is both depressed and hostile, the negative emotions interact in a complex way to elevate inflammatory substances in the body. Anger and hostility trigger the production of immune proteins involved in inflammation called IL-6, which contribute to arterial plaque.[89]

In people who are prone to anger, hostility or revenge, studies using heart rate monitors have shown that their heart rate is in sympathetic overload. And in that constantly stimulated state, people are more prone to constricted arteries, high blood pressure and heart attack or stroke. *Anger kills.* Redford Williams, M.D. and Virginia Williams, Ph.D. wrote a book with the same name and offer 17 practical strategies to overcome hostile, cynical or aggressive behaviors.

The Hungry Heart

The great American author, John Steinbeck said, "A sad soul can kill you quicker than a germ." More women than men tend to become depressed, which increases their risk of vascular disease. Depressed people are more likely to smoke, overeat or drink too much alcohol, and are less likely to keep active, promoting obesity and perpetuating depression.[90] The anonymity and loss of community in our society are key factors in the rise of vascular disease. Study after study show that people who feel lonely and depressed are more likely to get sick and die prematurely than those who have a strong connection to a caring community.[91] The heart is nourished by relationships with other people. Loneliness and isolation are *real* risk factors. Social and cultural factors have powerful effects on vascular functioning.

Even owning a dog or cat can help keep your blood pressure in check. Oxytocin, a neurochemical that lowers blood pressure, heart rate and the stress hormone, cortisol, normally rises during the interaction of people and their pets. Humans with higher oxytocin levels are more resistant to stress and more likely to trust other people.

Depression is especially hard on the heart. Cardiac rehabilitation patients who have symptoms of depression take longer to return to their normal heart rate after taking a treadmill stress test. Heart rate recovery after exercise is an indication of how well the autonomic nervous system functions. Patients who take longer to recover their normal heart rate have an increased risk of mortality.[92] Depression, like any form of pain, is a sign that we need to change the way we're doing something, and transform our lives for the better.

Food as Medicine

People experiencing depression or anxiety may have lowered dopamine levels in the brain. Pleasurable behavior such as eating, drinking and having sex increase brain dopamine levels, which explains in part why depression can lead to addictions. Areas of the brain responsible for memory and sensing pleasure are partially to blame. The neurobiology of compulsive overeating is similar to other addictions.

Many people who are addicted to foods share addictions to alcohol, tobacco and drugs. Substance abuse appears to work by mimicking key neurochemicals in the brain related to mood and pleasure. For example, nicotine binds to the receptors for the neurotransmitter, acetylcholine. Chocolate contains caffeine, an amphetamine-like ingredient that acts like an opiate by stimulating endorphins and other mediators in the brain. Eating cake, pizza, ice cream and other confectionery delights stimulates our bodies' release of natural opiates, the powerful relatives of morphine. If you're susceptible to binging, trying eating small meals throughout the day to prevent hunger, and be sure to have only small amounts of your desired food on hand.

Food cravings can also surface to satisfy hormonal deficits. Women who crave high-carbohydrate, salty or sugary foods just before their periods may be experiencing estrogen withdrawal. Following a low-fat, high-fiber diet, like the complex carbohydrate Non-Diet, can significantly reduce estrogen levels and help balance these hormonal changes.[93]

Food can be a powerful anti-depressant. Consuming wholesome complex carbohydrates appeases depression by increasing the brain passage of tryptophan, an essential amino acid and the precursor of serotonin, a neurotransmitter that counterbalances depression and obsessive-compulsive behavior, including overeating. Sticking to a Non-Dieting way of life for at least six weeks can help resolve food addictions and compulsive eating behaviors that can lead to obesity and vascular disease. A stomach full of high-carbohydrate, low fat foods can curb the tendency to cheat yourself out of great mental, emotional and physical health.

Open Mind, Open Heart

In my position as a neurosurgeon, I have spent years learning to have an open mind, and even longer striving to have an open heart. When the reasons for patients' visits to physicians are examined, about 75 percent of visits are related to stress and other psychosocial factors.[94]

Today, when I examine patients, I try to look into their hearts as much as their minds.

THE HEART SPEAKS

In her book *The Heart Speaks*, cardiologist Mimi Guarneri, M.D. laments that cardiologists today often act like "high-tech plumbers, more trained to sit and wait for someone to have a heart attack than to prevent one from happening." When describing her experience in medical school, Dr. Guarneri notes:

> No one spoke of the other layers of the heart that didn't appear on a stress test or electrocardiogram: the mental heart, affected by hostility, stress, and depression, the emotional heart that could be crushed by loss, the intelligent heart that has a nervous system of its own and communicates with the brain and other parts of the body.

Americans spend $18 billion annually on heart disease with an average cost of $50,000 for open-heart surgery or $10,000 for an angiogram. If we followed a more thoughtful approach to medical care, we could avoid overtreatment. As Dr. Ornish would say, surgery bypasses the problem. "It's a little like mopping the floor under a leaky sink without turning off the faucet. Sometimes you have to mop the floor, but if you don't turn off the faucet, the problem comes back again."[95] Dr. Ornish believes that heart patients can only fully recover by intimately opening their hearts through support groups that have stress-relief and healing that benefits a healthy lifestyle.

Pre-wired for Positive Emotions

It is important to remember that your mind and body are connected. The heart and brain communicate through the nervous system and chemical messengers. Strong emotions can cause the release of epinephrine and other hormones that increase heart rate and blood pressure. You not only deal with emotions of the moment, but also with an accumulation of experiences in your emotional memory banks. Emotions, pain and memory are deeply intertwined in your mind body.

The collective stress generated from negative feelings, thoughts and memories can be very damaging to your body. Amplified and reinforced through TV, radio and print media, the momentum for emotional stress is global, reaching billions of people daily. What we hear broadcast daily, murder, terrorism, war and natural disasters, impacts our thoughts and moods and we remain connected with that negative information.

The amygdala, an almond-shaped region in the brain, processes and imprints highly emotional memories. Infants are born with a well-developed amygdala, which is why a baby cries when picked up by an unfamiliar person or taken to an unfamiliar place. Fear is a primitive survival tactic. Autistics have a highly-reduced amygdala. They are unable to process several emotions, including the comprehension of fear or aggression in people's faces or behavioral expressions. The amygdala assigns emotional significance to everything you hear, smell, touch and see. Your perceptions of the environment and those around you travel directly to the amygdala without passing through the frontal cortex, the area that involves your ability to recognize future consequences resulting from current actions. You feel before you think. In dangerous situations, when you need to act fast, you can thank your amygdala.

Your earliest memories are usually emotion-laden. Do you remember the first time you touched a hot surface? Fear is a learned response. People who suffer traumatic experiences can develop overwhelming memories. The "fight or flight" rush of adrenaline cements especially sticky, almost obsessive memories. Highly stressful memories are stored in your brain's amygdala, and may not be accessible to your conscious mind. Memories of emotional experiences can influence the way we feel and behave beyond our awareness, protecting us from danger but also causing unconscious stress.

Fortunately, unconscious stress, anxiety and depression are treatable with psychotherapy, yoga, meditation or even getting up and getting out for a walk on a regular basis. Sometimes medications like antidepressants can help too.

Herbert Benson, M.D., who became well-known through his work on the stress response, believes that our bodies are genetically hardwired to benefit from our rich inner core of beliefs, values, thoughts and feelings. Social neuroscientists claim that "mirror neurons" may explain character traits or dispositions that equip people for success with interpersonal relationships including empathy, kindness, faith, generosity, trust and forgiveness.

The human brain has multiple mirror neuron systems which specialize in performing and understanding, not just the movement of others but their intentions and the social and emotional meaning of their behavior. Human relationships shape the brain's neural connections. According to Daniel Goleman in *Social Intelligence*, "Mirror neurons offer a neural mechanism that explains emotional contagion, the tendency of one person to catch the feelings of another, particularly if strongly expressed."[96] Neuroscientists and psychologists think that mirror neurons allow us to grasp the minds of others through intuition, not by thinking. If you see someone lose their temper or cry, mirror neurons in your brain simulate the distress. You are pre-wired to feel how others feel.[97]

Negative emotions and inflexible mindsets only put you in a state of emotional and physical incoherence that not only affects you, but those around you, especially children and pets. Have you ever noticed that a pet becomes more aggressive when someone in the room is arguing?

Psychological stress is one of the strongest predictors of future vascular events. Anger, depression, hostility and anxiety strongly contribute to vascular disease, stroke, heart attack and sudden cardiac death. Regulating these emotional states is as important as monitoring inflammation, cholesterol, blood pressure and sugar levels. With stress only increasing in the world, we need to go on the defensive with relaxation techniques, exercise, good relationships and disease-fighting foods to counter the devastating and often surprising complications of vascular disease.

Recommended Reading

In his book, *Eat More, Weigh Less,* Dr. Ornish offers 250 delicious low-fat, high fiber recipes for people who want to lose weight and improve their health. *The New McDougal Cookbook* offers 300 vegan high-carbohydrate and virtually fat-free recipes for people who want to reverse vascular disease and regain their health. Another program that follows the rules of Non-Dieting is Caldwell Esselstyn, Jr., M.D.'s *Prevent and Reverse Heart Disease.* There are other books that offer recipes with nutrient-dense foods but these three are specifically to reverse or prevent vascular disease. The recipes follow the high-fiber, low-fat complex carb way of eating, the Non-Diet. The diet plans in Dr. Fuhrman's *Eat to Live* claim to give obese people the opportunity to lose 15 to 25 pounds per month, with menus and recipes included.

Mind Body Science

Welcome To Your Mind Body, Mind Your Body Mend Your Health by Rudy Kachmann, M.D. & Kim Kachmann-Geltz, M.A.
The Second Brain by Michael D. Gershon, M.D.
Molecules of Emotion, The Science Behind Mind-Body Medicine by Candace Pert, Ph.D.
Anatomy of an Illness as Perceived by the Patient by Norman Cousins
The Relaxation Response by Herbert Benson
Love, Medicine & Miracles by Bernie Siegel

Cancer Recovery

Welcome To Your Mind Body, Mind Your Body Mend Your Health by Rudy Kachmann, M.D. & Kim Kachmann-Geltz, M.A.
Getting Well Again by O. Carl Simonton, M.D., Stephanie Matthews-Simonton, & James Creighton
The Will to Live by Arnold Hutschnecker, M.D.
Peace, Love, & Healing by Bernie Siegel, M.D.
Cancer as a Turning Point, Revised Edition by Lawrence LeShan, Ph.D.
Love, Medicine & Miracles by Bernie Siegel
Mind as Healer Mind as Slayer by Kenneth Pelletier
Beating Cancer with Nutrition by Patrick Quillen, Ph.D., R.D., C.N.S.

Fighting Cancer from Within by Martin L. Rossman, M.D.
9 Steps for Reversing or Preventing Cancer and Other Diseases by Shivani Goodman, Ed.D.

Wellness

The Stress of Life by Hans Selye
Molecules of Emotion, The Science Behind Mind-Body Medicine by Candace Pert, Ph.D.
Timeless Healing by Herbert Benson
How to Live 365 Days a Year by John Schindler, M.D.
Tension Myositis by John Sarno
Recovery Yoga by Sam Dworkis
Relax and Renew: Restful Yoga for Stressful Times by Judith Lasater
Meditation as Medicine by Dharma Singh Khalsa, M.D., & Cameron Stauth
Complete Book of Chinese Health and Healing, Guarding the Three Treasures by Daniel P. Reid
Guided Imagery for Self-Healing: An Essential Resource for Anyone Seeking Wellness by Martin L. Rossman
Fibromyalgia and the MindBody Spirit Connection: 7 Steps for Living a Healthy Life with Widespread Muscular Pain and Fatigue by William Bradley Salt & Edwin H. Season
The Acupuncture Response: Balance Energy and Restore Health - A Western Doctor Tells You How by Glenn S. Rothfeld & Suzanne LeVert
Eight Weeks to Optimum Health: A Proven Program for Taking Full Advantage of your Body's Natural Healing Power by Andrew Weil
Natural Health, Natural Medicine: The Complete Guide to Wellness and Self-Care for Optimum Health by Andrew Weil
The Easy Way to Stop Smoking by Allen Carr
Healing Back Pain: The Mind-Body Connection by Dr. John Sarno

Yoga, Meditation & Mindfulness

Full Catastrophe Living by Jon Kabat-Zinn, Ph.D.
Kundalini Yoga: The Flow of Eternal Power by Shakti Parwha Kaur Khalsa
YOGA For Transformation by Gary Kraftsow
Anatomy of Hatha Yoga: A Manual for Students, Teachers, and Practitioners by David Coulter
The Everyday Meditator: A Practical Guide by Osho

Creative Visualization Meditations by Shakti Gawain

The Heart of Yoga: Developing a Personal Practice by T.K.V. Desikachar

Light on Yoga: The Bible of Modern Yoga... by B.K.S. Iyengar

A Path with Heart: A Guide Through the Perils and Promises of Spiritual Life by Jack Kornfield

The Sevenfold Journey: Reclaiming Mind, Body & Spirit Through the Chakras by Judith and Vega

Structural Yoga Therapy: Adapting to the Individual by Mukunda Stiles

Yoga for Your Type: An Ayurvedic Approach to Your Asana Practice by Dr. David Frawley & Sandra Summerfield Rozak M.S.

Book Yourself Solid by Michael Port

Cool Yoga Tricks by Miriam Austin

Dancing the Body of Light by Donna Hollemann

Guiding Yoga's Light: Yoga Lessons for Yoga Teachers by Nancy Gerstein

Wherever You Go, There You Are: Mindfulness Meditation in Everyday Life by Zinn

Yoga for the Three Stages of Life: Developing Your Practice As an Art Form, a Physical Therapy, and a Guiding Philosophy by Ramaswami

Yoga for Wellness: Healing with the Timeless Teachings of Viniyoga by Kraftsow

Yoga of Heart: The Healing Power of Intimate Connection by Mark Whitwell

Yoga: The Iyengar Way by Mehta

Stress Management

Managing Stress: Principles and Strategies for Health and Wellbeing by Brian Luke Seaward

Will Yoga and Meditation Really Change My Life? American Teachers Share Their Stories by Stephen Cope

Nutrition & Health

The Secret of the Non-Diet to Prevent or Reverse Vascular Disease by Rudy Kachmann, M.D. & Kim Kachmann-Geltz, M.A.

Eat More Weigh Less by Dr. Dean Ornish

Eat To Live by Joel Fuhrman, M.D.

The China Study by T. Colin Campbell, Ph.D & Thomas M. Campbell II

Dr. Attwood's Low-Fat Prescription of Kids by Charles R. Attwood
Prevent and Reverse Heart Disease by Caldwell B. Esselstyn
Take a Load off Your Heart by Joeseph C. Piscatella & Barry Franklin
McDougall Program for Maximum Weight Loss by John A. McDougall &
    Mary A. McDougall
Reversing Heart Disease by Julian Whitaker, M.D.
Eating Well for Optimum Health by Andrew Weil

Acknowledgments

The co-author would like to first thank her father for changing the way she looks at food. (I hope it's not too late). I would also like to thank my family—Scott, Jessica, Samantha, Coulson, Mom, Jeff, Belinda, Heidi, Will—for the many sacrifices they made while Dad and I were writing this book. I may never be a cook but I hope you can see now that my love is for the pen.

END NOTES

[1] Walter Willett, M.D., Fredrick John Stare Professor of Epidemiology and Nutrition, Harvard School of Public Health, and professor of medicine, Harvard Medical School, Boston.

[2] National Center for Health Statistics, *National Vital Statistics Reports*; 53: 17; 2005.

[3] "Role of inflammation—Growing proof inflammation is a major risk factor for heart disease," Cleveland Clinic Heart & Vascular Institute Web site, August, 2002.

[4] P.M. Ridker, et al., "Comparison of C-Reactive Protein and Low-Density Lipoprotein Cholesterol Levels in the Prediction of First Cardiovascular Events," *New England Journal of Medicine*, 347:1557; 2002.

[5] Mora, S., et al., "Physical Activity and Reduced Risk of Cardiovascular Events: Potential Mediating Mechanisms," *Circulation*; 116: 2110 – 2118; 2007.

[6] Campbell, T. Colin, *The China Study: The Most Comprehensive Study of Nutrition Ever Conducted and the Startling Implications for Diet, Weight Loss and Long-term Health*, Benbella Books, 2006.

[7] Nissen, Steven E., M.D., et al., *The New England Journal of Medicine*, 352:29; 2005.

[8] Ornish, D., et al., "Can lifestyle changes reverse coronary heart disease? The Lifestyle Heart Trial," *Lancet*; Jul 21; 336 (8708):129-33; 1990.

[9] Esselstyn, Caldwell B., Jr., *Prevent and Reverse Heart Disease*, Avery, 2007.

[10] Centers for Disease Control and Prevention, National Health Center for Statistics, "Obesity Still a Major Problem," April 14, 2006.

[11] Convit, A., "Hypothalamic-Pituitary-Adrenal Axis Dysregulation and Memory Impairments in Type 2 diabetes," *The Journal of Clinical Endocrinology & Metabolism*; Vol. 92, No. 7 2439-2445; 2007.

[12] Zhang, C., et al., "Abdominal Obesity and the Risk of All-Cause, Cardiovascular, and Cancer Mortality: Sixteen Years of Follow-Up in US Women," *Circulation*, Apr 2008; 117: 1658 - 1667.

[13] Pollan, M., "Unhappy Meals," *The New York Times Magazine*, January 28, 2007.

[14] Ibid, Campbell, C.

[15] World Health Organization, Joint WHO/FAO Expert Consultation "Diet, Nutrition and the Prevention of Chronic Diseases," WHO Technical Report Series 916; 2003.

[16] Chandalia M. et al., "Beneficial effects of high dietary fiber intake in patients with type 2 diabetes mellitus," *New England Journal of Medicine*; 342:1392-1398; 2000.

[17] Slyper, A., "Influence of glycemic load on HDL cholesterol in youth," *American Journal of Clinical Nutrition*; 81: 2, 376-379; 2005.

[18] Jacobs, D., *American Journal of Clinical Nutrition*; 68: 248, 1998.

[19] Pollan, Michael, *In Defense of Food*, Penguin Press, 2008.

[20] Aviram M, Rosenblat M, Gaitini D, et al, "Pomegranate juice consumption for 3 years by patients with carotid artery stenosis reduces common carotid intima-media thickness, blood pressure and LDL oxidation," *Clin Nutr* 23 (3): 423–33; June, 2004.

[21] Studer, M., "Effect of Different Antilipidemic Agents and Diets on Mortality: A Systematic Review," *The Archives of Internal Medicine*; 165:725 – 730; 2005.

[22] AP, Simopoulos, "Omega-3 fatty acids in health and disease and in growth and development," *Am J Clin Nutr*; 54:438-63; 1991.

[23] Katan MB, et al., "Trans fatty acids and their effects on lipoproteins in humans," *Annual Review of Nutrition*; 15:473-93; 1995.

[24] Rafferty, J., "Trans Fat 'Ban Wagon,'" *Harvard Public Health Review*, http://www.hsph.harvard.edu/review/spring07/spr07transfat.html; 2007.

[25] Ascherio A, Stampfer MJ, Willett WC, "Trans fatty acids and coronary heart disease," Harvard School of Public Health, http://www.hsph.harvard.edu/; 2006.

[26] Wilson, M., "Carbohydrates, Proteins, and Fats," *Merck Manual of Medical Information*, http://www.merck.com/mmhe/print/sec12/ch152/ch152b.html; 2008.

[27] Pischon, T., *The New England Journal of Medicine*; 359:2105-2120; 2008.

[28] Ibid, Willett, W.

[29] U.S. Department of Agriculture, *Economic Research Service Briefing*, May 25, 2007.

[30] Fleming, R., "The effect of high-protein diets on coronary blood flow," *Angiography*; 51 (10):817-26; 2000.

[31] Ibid, Campbell.

[32] Ob cit, Campbell.

[33] Kuo, P., "Angina pectoris induced by fat ingestion in patients with coronary artery disease," *Journal of the American Medical Association*; 1008-1013; July 23, 1955.

[34] Esselstyn, C., "Resolving the Coronary Artery Disease Epidemic through Plant-Based Nutrition," *Preventative Cardiology*; 4: 171-177; 2001.

[35] Tsai AG, Wadden, et al., "Systematic review: an evaluation of major commercial weight loss programs in the United States," *Annals of Internal Medicine*; 142 (1):56-66; 2005.

[36] Dansinger ML et al., "Comparison of the Atkins, Ornish, Weight Watchers and Zone diets for weight loss and heart disease risk reduction: a randomized trial,: *JAMA* ;293: 43–53; 2005.

[37] Brownell, K., "Fighting Obesity and the Food Lobby," *The Washington Post*, June 9, 2002; Page B07.

[38] CDC, National Center for Health Statistics, National Health and Nutrition Examination Survey, *Journal of the American Medical Association*, 2002; 288:1723-7; 2002.

[39] Olshansky, J., "A Potential Decline in Life Expectancy in the United States in the 21st Century," *New England Journal of Medicine*; 352:1138-1145; 2005.

[40] Deakin University; "Study Shows Fruit Juice/Drink Link to Children's Weight Gain," *Science Daily*, 29 March 2007.

[41] Libby, P., "Atherosclerosis: the New View," *Scientific Am.*; 286 (5):46-55; May; 2002.

[42] Libby, P., "The molecular mechanisms of the thrombotic complications of atherosclerosis," *Journal of Internal Medicine*; 263(5):517-27; May 2008.

[43] P.M. Ridker, et al., "C-reactive protein and other markers of inflammation in the prediction of cardiovascular disease in women," *New England Journal of Medicine*, 342(12):836-43, 2000.

[44] Robinson, Joshua, "After Completing Marathon, a Runner Dies in His Home," *The New York Times*, November 7, 2007.

[45] Kandel, E., *In Search of Memory: The Emergence of a New Science of Mind*, W.W. Norton, 2007.

[46] Garrison, Julia Fox, *Don't Leave Me This Way*, Harper Collins, 2007.

[47] Cheng, M., "Studies Tout Treating Mini-Strokes Fast," *Brain in the News*, November 2007.

[48] Ibid, Cheng.

[50] Women and cardiovascular diseases statistics, American Heart Association, 2004.

[51] Kolata, G., "Reversing Trend, Big Drop Is Seen in Breast Cancer," *The New York Times*, December 15, 2006.

[52] Miller, A.P, et al., "Secondary Prevention of Coronary Heart Disease in Women: A Call to Action," *Annals of Internal Medicine*; 138 2 81-160; 2001.

[53] Cook, N., et al., "Physical Activity and Reduced Risk of Cardiovascular Events: Potential Mediating Mechanisms," *Circulation: Journal of the American Heart Association*; 116: 2110 – 2118; 2007.

[54] P. Barberger-Gateau, et al., "Dietary patterns and risk of dementia," *Neurology*, 69:1921-1930; 2007.

[55] Morris, Martha C.; Sacks, Frank; Rosner, Bernard, Does fish oil lower blood pressure? A meta-analysis of controlled trials," *Circulation*; 88 (2): 523–533; 1993.

[56] Sanders, T., et al., "Influence of n–6 versus n–3 polyunsaturated fatty acids in diets low in saturated fatty acids on plasma lipoproteins and hemostatic factors," *Arteriosclerosis, Thrombosis, and Vascular Biology*; 17 (12): 3449–3460; 1997.

[57] National Health and Nutrition Examination Survey (NHANES), 1999-2004, National Center for Health Statistics and the NHLBI.

[58] Esselstyn, C., *Prevent and Reverse Heart Disease*, Penguin Group, 2007.

[59] Whitaker, Julian, *Reversing Heart Disease*, Warner Books, 2002.

[60] Levy, R., "Report on the Lipid Research Clinic Trials," *European Heart Journal*, E: 45-53; August 1987.

[61] Flegal, K., et al., "Cause-specific excess deaths associated with underweight, overweight, and obesity," *Journal of American Medical Association*; 298: 2028-2037; 2007.

[62] *American College of Radiology* press release, "Zoos Stretched to Limit as Providers Seek Supersized Scanners for Morbidly Obese Patients," 2008.

[63] Frazao, E. et al., "America's eating habits: changes and consequences," USDA/ERS Agri. Info. Bull. 750; 1999.

[64] Cutler, D., et al., "Why Have Americans Become More Obese?" *The Economics of Obesity*; Economic Research Service/USDA.

[65] Wilson, P. et al., *Archives of Internal Medicine*; 162: 1867-1872; 2002.

[66] Ezzati, M., et al., "Causes of cancer in the world: comparative risk assessment of nine behavioral and environmental risk factors," *The Lancet*; 366:1784–1793; 2005.

[67] Lutsey, P., "Dietary Intake and the Development of the Metabolic Syndrome," *Circulation*; 117:754-761; 2008.

[68] "Dietary Intake and the Development of the Metabolic Syndrome," *Circulation*; 117:754-761; 2008.

[69] "Pre-diabetes," Mayo Clinic.com, Jan. 5, 2008.

[70] Kaufman, F., *Diabesity*, Bantam Books, 2005.

[71] National Diabetes Statistics; National Institutes for Health; 2005.

[72] Ibid, Kaufman, F.

[73] Brody, Jane E., "'Diabesity,' a Crisis in an Expanding Country," *The New York Times*, March 29, 2005.

[74] Jensen, M., "Intakes of whole grains, bran, and germ and the risk of coronary heart disease in men," *American Journal of Clinical Nutrition*; 80: 6, 1492-1499; 2004.

[75] Sachiko, T., et al., Statement of the AHA Nutrition Committee; *Circulation*; 104:1869; 2001.

[76] "Reduction of Type 2 Diabetes with Lifestyle Interventions," *New England Journal of Medicine*; 346: 393-403; 2002.

[77] "Long-term Effects of Renin-Angiotensin System–Blocking Therapy and a Low Blood Pressure Goal on Progression of Hypertensive Chronic Kidney Disease in African-Americans," *Arch Intern Med.*; 168(8):832-839; 2008.

[78] 10 ways to control high blood pressure without medication, MayoClinic.com, May 21, 2008.

[79] Flack, J., "Epidemiology of Hypertension and Cardiovascular Disease in African-Americans," *The Journal of Clinical Hypertension*; Volume 5 Issue 1 Page 5-11; 2003.

[80] Benjamin EJ, et al., "Evidence-Based Guidelines for Cardiovascular Disease Prevention in Women: 2007 Update," *Circulation*; 2007.

[81] Fuhrman, Joel, *Eat to Live*, Little, Brown, & Co., 2003.

[82] High Blood Pressure Statistics, American Heart Association.org, 2008.

[83] Guimont, C., et al., "Chronic job strain may raise blood pressure," *American Journal of Public Health*, August 2006.

[84] Ruiz, J., et al., "Association between muscular strength and mortality in men: prospective cohort study," *British Medical Journal*; 337:a439;2008.

[85] Didion, J., *The Year of Magical Thinking*, Knopf, 2005.

[86] Bajaj, V. "An Enron Chapter Closes: An Obituary; Kenneth L. Lay, 64, Enron Founder and Symbol of Corporate Excess," *The New York Times*, July 5, 2006.

[87] Shedd, O., et al., "The World Trade Center attack: Increased frequency of defibrillator shocks for ventricular arrhythmias in patients living remotely from New York City," *Journal of the American College of Cardiology*; vol. 44: 6, pp. 1265-1267; 2004.

[88] Guarneri, M., *The Heart Speaks*, Touchstone, 2006.

[89] Lavelle, P. "Anger trigger to heart disease found?" *ABC Science Online*, 2003.

[90] World Health Organization, "The World Health Report 2001: Mental Health: New Understanding, New Hope."

[91] Nielsen, KM, "Danish singles have a twofold risk of acute coronary syndrome," *Journal of Epidemiology and Community Health*; 60:721-728; 2006.

[92] Hughes, J., *American Heart Journal*, May 2006.

[93] Bagga D, et al., "Effects of a very low fat, high fiber diet on serum hormones and menstrual function," *Cancer*; 76:2491-6; 1995.

[94] Gureje, O., et al., "Persistent Pain and Well-being: A World Health Organization Study in Primary Care," *Journal of American Medical Association*, 280(2): 147-51, 1998.

[95] Ornish, D., "Love Is Real Medicine," *Newsweek*, October 3, 2005.

[96] Goleman, D., *Social Intelligence: The New Science of Human Relationships*, Bantam, 2006.

[97] Blakeslee, S., "Cells that Read Minds," *The New York Times*, January 10, 2006.

ABOUT THE AUTHORS

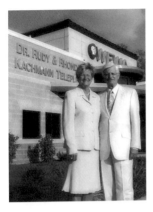

Rudy Kachmann, M.D., is the cofounder of the Kachmann Mind Body Institute in Fort Wayne, Indiana, and has been in practice for over 40 years. Dr. Kachmann received his Neurosurgery training from Georgetown University. He received his M.D. and a B.S. in Chemistry from Indiana University.

His major interests are wellness and holistic healing. He has been on PBS and his lectures have been broadcast on PBS. He is a regular lecturer on subjects of the mind body including diet, stress, cancer, back pain and Asian healing. He lectures to corporations and includes stress and finances lectures. He is regularly featured in local media, including radio shows, doing a regular monthly television broadcast called "Docs on Call," newspapers, magazines and medical journals. He is the author of *Twenty Prescriptions for Living the Good Life, Welcome to Your Mind Body*, DVDs on mind body, back pain, a DVD lecture series and producer of *Oh My Aching Back*.

Dr. Kachmann is on the Board of Directors of Day Break Children's Shelter and the Board of Trustees of Lutheran Hospital. He is the founder of the Kachmann Behavioral Foundation that funds community-based educational initiatives, and is a member of the Tennis Hall of Fame. He has received several awards, including the Martin Luther King award for his support of community outreach. Dr. Kachmann is a long-time resident of Fort Wayne where he lives with his wife, Yorkshire terrier and two Tonkinese cats.

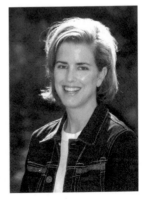

Kim Kachmann-Geltz received a B.A. in humanities from Indiana University and a M.A. in American Studies from Columbia University. Her writing career began as a legislative correspondent on Capitol Hill. Her knowledge of health care and medicine grew as the director of SpeakOutUSA, a non-profit that developed educational videos and produced health care reform hearings for bipartisan members of the U.S. Congress.

She joined America Online, Inc. as writer and editor of the "Welcome Screen" before becoming director of AOL International Content & Programming. There she developed the company's first manual on editorial content standards, practices and taught the "best practices" to AOL's joint ventures in 11 different countries around the world.

She lives on Hilton Head Island with her husband, three young children, Yorkshire terrier, rabbit and two Tonkinese cats.

The Kachmann Mind Body Institute is the leader in research, education, and clinical practice of mind body medicine. We teach various complementary mind body therapies as the ultimate integrative and holistic approach to healing. We recognize the connection between human experience, self awareness and one's health. Not only are we interested in helping build a healthy immune system, but we are interested in helping build a healthy mind. We help individuals understand how the mind and body are interconnected and how they function as a whole.

The Kachmann Mind Body Institute is dedicated to helping individuals create and maintain lifelong health through various mind body programs including:

- Group Yoga & Fitness Classes & Workshops
- Weight Management
- Personal Fitness Training
- Holistic Pain Management
- Yoga Therapy
- Massage Therapy
- Corporate Wellness
- Dr. Rudy Kachmann Lecture Series
- Physician Consultation

Lutheran Hospital Campus
7900 West Jefferson Blvd.
Suite 108 MOB1
Fort Wayne, IN 46804

Downtown Fort Wayne
1301 Layette St.
Suite 205
Fort Wayne, IN 46802

For more information please contact us at 260-420-YOGA (9642) or visit www.KachmannMindBody.com